Not Rocket Science

Not Rocket Science

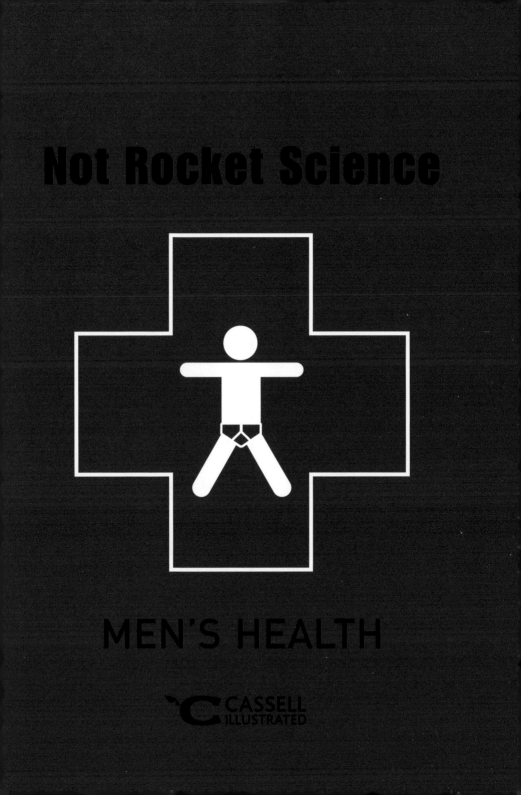

MEN'S HEALTH

CASSELL
ILLUSTRATED

FIRST PUBLISHED IN GREAT BRITAIN IN 2005 BY CASSELL ILLUSTRATED,
A DIVISION OF OCTOPUS PUBLISHING GROUP LIMITED
2–4 HERON QUAYS, LONDON E14 4JP

CONCEPT, EDITORIAL, DESIGN AND LAYOUT BY ESSENTIAL WORKS LTD.
168A CAMDEN STREET, LONDON NW1 9PT, ENGLAND

DISTRIBUTED IN THE UNITED STATES OF AMERICA BY
STERLING PUBLISHING CO., INC.,
387 PARK AVENUE SOUTH, NEW YORK, NY 10016-8810

A CIP CATALOGUE RECORD FOR THIS BOOK IS AVAILABLE FROM THE BRITISH LIBRARY.

ISBN 1 84403 270 1
EAN 9781844032709

PRINTED IN CHINA

Because we can't all be like Keith,

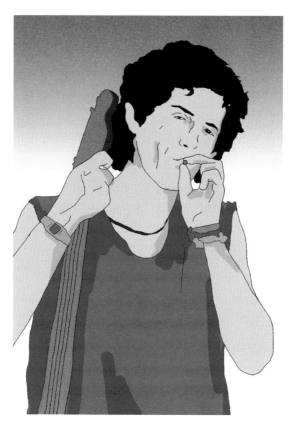

Contents

Booze (and drugs) 148

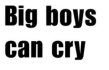

Big boys
can cry   170

6

The ages of man

7

Whaddya mean, you've never worried about your health?

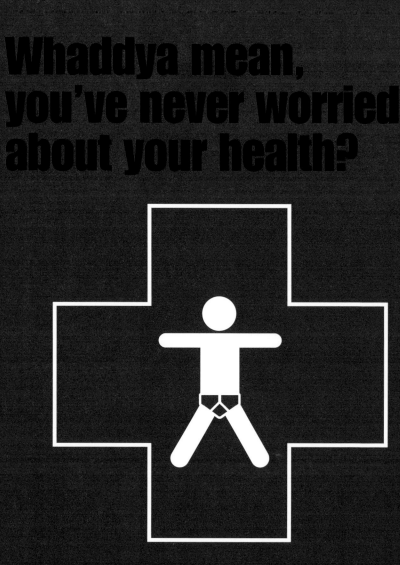

THE TROUBLE WITH BAD HEALTH IS YOU NEVER KNOW WHEN IT'S GOING TO HIT YOU, OR HOW, OR, COME TO THAT, WHAT PART OF YOUR BODY IT'S GOING TO AFFECT. UNLESS, OF COURSE, YOU'RE WOBBLING WITH FAT OR HAVE BEEN A 60-A-DAY SMOKER FOR THE LAST TEN YEARS – THEN YOU'LL HAVE A FAIR IDEA THAT IT'LL BE EITHER YOUR HEART OR YOUR LUNGS. BUT THE POINT IS, AS MEN, WE OUGHT TO BE BETTER PREPARED FOR WHAT LIFE MIGHT THROW AT US. HELL – BEING PREPARED AT ALL WOULD BE A START.

It's a fact that, in spite of awareness campaigns by governments and a growing bookshelf available on the subject of men's health, very few of us know much about it beyond testicular cancer. Through a combination of fear and sheer bone idleness, we don't bother to find out anything that isn't relevant to us at any particular time because we don't like not being in control of our destiny and we've got far more important things to do. In other words, we'll make any excuse not to go to the doctor and will never take health matters as seriously as our wives (who have turned them into some sort of hobby).

More fool us. And we're only fooling ourselves, too, because we're never in so much control of our lives that we can't take advice from an expert, the GP. How in control will you be when you're gasping for air or stretched out on an operating table? As for being too busy to take care of ourselves,

'Always put a dead weasel on a broken ankle'

Some facts and fictions of men's health:

An apple a day keeps the doctor away.
You're lucky to get a doctor who does house calls – but eating today's hydroponic, nutrient-lacking, engineered-to-look-good-in-the-supermarket apples won't do you much good at all. Just eat more fruit.

You don't catch cold from being cold.
In spite of what your mum always told you, a cold is a viral infection.

There is no such thing as a wig that 'nobody will notice'.
Why do people bother? Surely being seen as a slaphead can't be as humiliating as having perfect strangers snigger at your rug?

Research has shown that wearing Y-fronts does not inhibit your fertility.
It might not help your ability to find somebody who wants her eggs fertilised by you, though.

Low-fat foods aren't necessarily good for you.
It's all in the wording – 15 per cent fat free means the rest could be 85 per cent fat. And 'low' or 'lower' fat is comparing it to what? Always read the small labels as well as the big ones.

Women are the weaker sex.
Wrong. They live longer, are less susceptible to a lot of illnesses and less likely to have drink problems.

we'd function that much better if we were at peak health and fitness. Who will 'get the job done' when you're in hospital? The trick to remember is the one that women have known for years: make the effort to look after yourself as a matter of course, and you'll be that much less likely to need looking after by somebody else later on. Now how in control is that?

This book is dedicated to preventive measures as much as it is to defensive action against something that's already happened. Go on the offensive against the conditions that could lead to serious ill-health. Lose weight! Take up running! Eat properly! Cut out binge drinking! These are all things that will vastly improve your quality of life as well as your health and longevity prospects. And they are actions that need to be taken now, more than ever before, as 21st-century living seems to be actively working against keeping men healthy.

Congratulations! By getting this far into this book you are showing intelligence enough to live longer than the men who give up on listening to health advice as soon as they leave the clinic.

Know your history

A detailed knowledge of your family's medical history is vital for a better understanding of your own health, and a valuable asset to pass down to your children and their children. Many conditions are either hereditary or influenced by ancestry, so it will help you to spot the likelihood of certain illnesses if you know your grandfather or your great grandmother had them. And because the generations above you aren't going to be around for ever, it's important to get going on this as soon as possible.

Unless previous members of your family have kept written records, you are going to have to do some detective work. Start with your oldest living relatives and find out what they know about the health of those above and below them on the family tree. Then work your way down the tree towards yourself, asking the same questions. Ask people for their recollections of the generations in a different branch of the family from your own; somebody might remember something somebody else has forgotten. If you have children, get their mother to do the same thing.

Then write it all down. Draw a family tree connecting the different members of each generation, with box spaces for listing what conditions they had or what they might have been allergic to. Keep it in a safe place, updating it every time you get some new information, and make sure your children get copies of it.

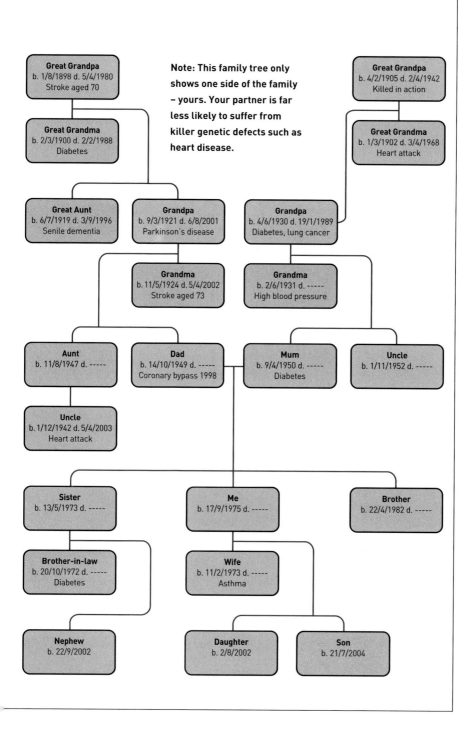

Great Grandpa
b. 1/8/1898 d. 5/4/1980
Stroke aged 70

Great Grandma
b. 2/3/1900 d. 2/2/1988
Diabetes

Note: This family tree only shows one side of the family – yours. Your partner is far less likely to suffer from killer genetic defects such as heart disease.

Great Grandpa
b. 4/2/1905 d. 2/4/1942
Killed in action

Great Grandma
b. 1/3/1902 d. 3/4/1968
Heart attack

Great Aunt
b. 6/7/1919 d. 3/9/1996
Senile dementia

Grandpa
b. 9/3/1921 d. 6/8/2001
Parkinson's disease

Grandpa
b. 4/6/1930 d. 19/1/1989
Diabetes, lung cancer

Grandma
b. 11/5/1924 d. 5/4/2002
Stroke aged 73

Grandma
b. 2/6/1931 d. -----
High blood pressure

Aunt
b. 11/8/1947 d. -----

Dad
b. 14/10/1949 d. -----
Coronary bypass 1998

Mum
b. 9/4/1950 d. -----
Diabetes

Uncle
b. 1/11/1952 d. -----

Uncle
b. 1/12/1942 d. 5/4/2003
Heart attack

Sister
b. 13/5/1973 d. -----

Me
b. 17/9/1975 d. -----

Brother
b. 22/4/1982 d. -----

Brother-in-law
b. 20/10/1972 d. -----
Diabetes

Wife
b. 11/2/1973 d. -----
Asthma

Nephew
b. 22/9/2002

Daughter
b. 2/8/2002

Son
b. 21/7/2004

Here, they are presented in a way that is as fun to read about as many of them are to do.

This book won't solve all your health problems; it's far from being a medical encyclopedia, but it can be much more important to your life than that. It is designed to start you off on that path to health.

There is a fitness saying that goes 'the only diets that work are the ones you stick to', and it's like that with health books: the only ones that do any good are the ones you want to read.

This book is user-friendly in the extreme – it won't patronise you, won't baffle you with medical terms or give you far too much knowledge to deal with. It will talk to you in a way you'll want to engage with and start you off on a road that leads to a new and much healthier you – a man who can really stay in control of his destiny.

Why you need to take your health more seriously

Ironically, although women devote more time and thought to their health than men, we really ought to be putting in the effort. When it comes to the sort of behaviour that can seriously damage our physical and emotional well-being, men are streets ahead. Men are much more likely to:

Smoke, and to smoke more cigarettes than women.

Although twentysomething women are doing their best to catch up, they've still got a way to go.

Drink heavily and binge drink.

Again, young women are holding their end up, but as they get older they will stop, whereas men are less likely to.

Be overweight or obese.

It just doesn't worry us like it does women.

Eat badly.

Men eat much more junk food and neglect the healthier options, which is doubtless related to the previous point.

Avoid going to the doctor.

Or confront anything that might be a medical problem.

Let stress affect their lives.

Women seem to be better natural multi-taskers and more able just to get on with it without letting things get them down – maybe because they cry more than we do.

Are you a hypochondriac?

Most men fear that if they take too much obvious interest in their health they'll be labelled hypochondriacs. But the truth is there's a yawning gulf between being concerned and fretting unnecessarily. Take our fun test and find out which side of the fence you are on. See page 16 to find out how you scored.

1 If you sneeze a couple of times during the course of a morning, and maybe blow your nose, what would be your likely reaction?
a 'Did I? I didn't notice.'
b 'Is there something going round?'
c 'Oh no, I could be going down with something.'
d 'Don't come near me. Not unless you've had a flu jab.'

2 Your medicine cabinet is:
a The drawer by the side of your bed, where an old box of aspirin lurks among the expired-date condoms and long-forgotten loose change.
b Half empty.
c Full of unfinished courses of prescribed tablets – well, you felt better, so you sort of forgot.
d In alphabetical order.

3 Your relationship with your doctor is:
a 'Who?'
b Only exists when a day or two in bed and a few paracetamol don't do the trick.
c Once a year for a check-up.
d You are on first-name terms with the receptionist.

4 A news item on a newly discovered strain of a well-known illness is:
a Nothing for you to worry about.
b Vaguely interesting.
c A good topic of conversation in the bar.
d A clear and present danger.

5 What's the difference between a migraine and a headache?
a A migraine is a hypochondriac's name for a headache.
b 'Isn't one much worse than the other?'
c Migraines may involve vomiting, disorientation, loss of balance, visual disturbances and adverse reaction to light; headaches make your head ache.
d 'I only have migraines.'

6 When on holiday do you drink the water?
a 'Who drinks water on holiday?'
b Once you've dropped in a couple of purifying tablets it's usually fine. Usually.
c Bottled water only.
d 'Don't let them put ice in your drinks or make you coffee because it all comes from the same water. And don't eat the fish either, they've been swimming in it.'

7 A trip to casualty is:
a A regular Friday night detour.
b A bloody nuisance – literally.
c A necessary evil.
d You can't be too sure about that dark patch on your arm.

8 How often and how rigorously do you feel your testicles?

a At every possible opportunity and with considerable enthusiasm; sometimes too much enthusiasm, or at least that's what the wife says.

b Usually when you're watching television, and it depends what's on.

c Once a month, probing gently round the testes for any abnormalities.

d At every possible opportunity, probing gently round the testes for any abnormalities.

9 When given advice on health, fitness and your lifestyle do you?

a Assume you are being confused with some sad bastard who has nothing else to do.

b Nod politely, smile, say thank you and promptly forget about it.

c Do your best to take it up because it seems to make sense.

d Put them right on a couple of points.

10 Why did you pick this book up?

a Your wife gave it to you and threatened no sex until you at least made some sort of effort.

b It looked like it might be an interesting read – a bit of a laugh.

c You've been meaning to do something about your health and fitness for quite a while now.

d It's the only men's health book you haven't got.

How did you score?

MOSTLY As

Hypochondriac Rating -10. It's a good thing you are actually reading this book, because your cavalier attitude to health will get you into all sorts of trouble once you are out of your teens.

MOSTLY Bs

Hypochondriac Rating -5. If you're older than your early thirties, you could have a few problems; although you're aware you're not invincible, you could be a bit more aware.

MOSTLY Cs

Hypochondriac Rating 0. You've hit a perfect balance between concern about your health and not letting it get in the way of your life.

MOSTLY Ds

Hypochondriac Rating 10. Your doctor must be getting sick of the sight of you and, besides, what's the point of being so healthy if it doesn't leave you the time to enjoy the benefits of it?

It really isn't rocket science

Men's health isn't really difficult, especially given that so much of what goes wrong with us is essentially self-inflicted. Lifestyles of the last couple of decades have done a great deal to change how healthy we are, and not much of it has been for the better. One of the themes this book keeps coming back to is how easy it is to do something about your health, and most of it is basic common sense.

STOP SMOKING

Lung cancer is one of the biggest killers in the UK, responsible for more deaths each year than road accidents, poisoning, murder, manslaughter, suicide and HIV combined, and it is inescapably linked to smoking. Worryingly, the rates of young men (under 35) smoking cigarettes are rising.

CUT DOWN ON YOUR DRINKING

Although it might not actually kill you, or if it does it will take a long time, heavy drinking is responsible for all sorts of men's health problems, not least the escalating levels of violence that are being perpetrated by young British men on other young British men in city centres every weekend.

GET SOME EXERCISE

Heart disease is another killer of Western men. As a nation, Britain is becoming progressively more obese and, as a result, rates of heart disease, high blood pressure, strokes and type 2 diabetes are dangerously on the rise. Regular aerobic exercise can go a long way to combating this.

EAT MORE FRESH FRUIT AND VEGETABLES

In recent times, the national diet has so deteriorated that malnutrition is frequently found to be the root cause of maladies among people who are convinced they are eating well. Processed foods should be substituted with fresh produce whenever possible.

WEAR SUN BLOCK IF YOU HAVE PALE SKIN

A few years ago a sun tan was believed to be the mark of good health, but it's more likely to be an overture for skin cancer. With the ozone layer being progressively depleted, everyone, and especially those with pale skin, needs to take extra care in the sun.

DON'T TREAT YOUR GP LIKE AN ALIEN

Too many men won't go to see their doctor if they don't feel well. It means that a great many health problems go undiagnosed until they are too serious to ignore.

♥ | 1 The heart of the matter

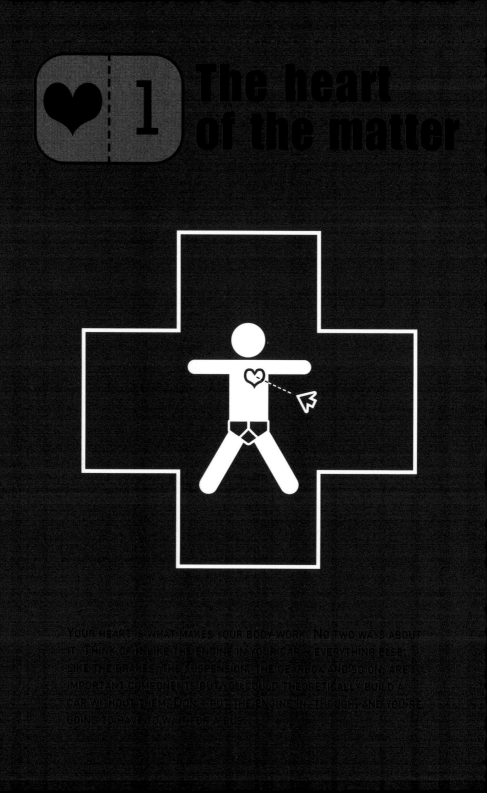

YOUR HEART IS WHAT MAKES YOUR BODY WORK. NO TWO WAYS ABOUT
IT. THINK OF IT LIKE THE ENGINE IN YOUR CAR. EVERYTHING ELSE,
LIKE THE BRAKES, THE SUSPENSION, THE GEARBOX AND SO ON, ARE
IMPORTANT COMPONENTS BUT YOU COULD THEORETICALLY BUILD A
CAR WITHOUT THEM. DON'T PUT THE ENGINE IN, THOUGH, AND YOU'RE
GOING TO HAVE TO WAIT FOR A BUS.

Like the beat-beat-beat of a tom-tom

A man's heart is about the size and shape of his clenched fist and is located behind the rib cage, a little to the left of centre. It is a powerful muscle, operating as a pump to move blood around the body and with it the oxygen and nutrients needed for sustaining life (see page 26). That is pretty much what everybody knows about the heart, but it's really a little more complicated.

Not only must the heart get the blood into circulation, but it must first pump it through the lungs to pick up oxygen and then receive the oxygenated blood back again before sending it on its way to every organ and tissue in the body. This operation is carried out through a simple yet highly sophisticated system comprising the four chambers (known as atria and ventricles) that divide the heart's hollow interior, and a series of one-way valves. Oxygen-depleted blood that has completed a circuit of the body drains into the right side of the heart via two large veins, the superior (upper) vena cava, which is connected to the upper body, and the inferior (lower) vena cava, which is connected to the lower body. Blood from both these channels flows into one of the heart's two upper chambers, known as the right atrium. From there the blood passes through three flaps of movable tissue, called the tricuspid valve, into one of the two lower chambers, the right ventricle. As it leaves this lower chamber, blood is pumped through another valve, the pulmonary valve, and into the pulmonary artery, which delivers it to the lungs.

Once it has collected oxygen in the lungs, this fresh blood returns from the lungs via the pulmonary veins to the heart. The process is pretty much repeated in reverse now. Oxygen-laden blood enters the upper left chamber (left atrium), passes through the

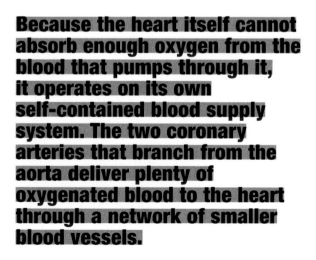

Because the heart itself cannot absorb enough oxygen from the blood that pumps through it, it operates on its own self-contained blood supply system. The two coronary arteries that branch from the aorta deliver plenty of oxygenated blood to the heart through a network of smaller blood vessels.

mitral valve down into the lower left chamber (left ventricle) and from there is pumped into the body's main artery, called the aorta, and so enters the circulatory system.

The four chambers of the heart are made of sheets of muscle containing fibres that contract and expand automatically to constitute the heart's beats. The upper chambers have much thinner walls than the lower chambers, and the left and right sides of the heart are separated by the septum, a strong wall of muscle that prevents oxygenated blood from mixing with deoxygenated blood. The heart has its own inbuilt pacemaker to regulate the speed and rhythm at which it pumps. A small clump of special tissue called the sinotrial node sends out impulses that make the upper chambers contract. This triggers impulses in another small clump, the atrioventricular (AV) node, situated in between the upper and lower chambers; in turn, the AV node passes on the message, making the muscle fibres of the lower chambers contract.

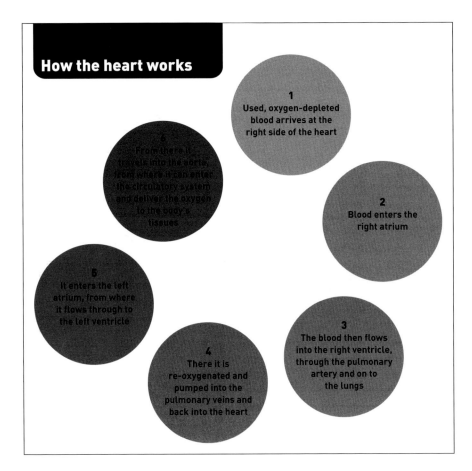

How the heart works

1 Used, oxygen-depleted blood arrives at the right side of the heart

2 Blood enters the right atrium

3 The blood then flows into the right ventricle, through the pulmonary artery and on to the lungs

4 There it is re-oxygenated and pumped into the pulmonary veins and back into the heart

5 It enters the left atrium, from where it flows through to the left ventricle

6 From there it travels into the aorta, from where it can enter the circulatory system and deliver the oxygen to the body's tissues

The heart

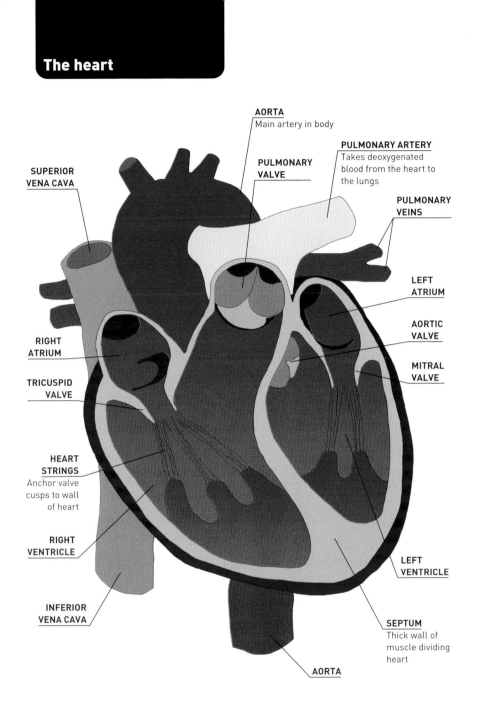

AORTA
Main artery in body

PULMONARY VALVE

PULMONARY ARTERY
Takes deoxygenated blood from the heart to the lungs

SUPERIOR VENA CAVA

PULMONARY VEINS

LEFT ATRIUM

AORTIC VALVE

RIGHT ATRIUM

MITRAL VALVE

TRICUSPID VALVE

HEART STRINGS
Anchor valve cusps to wall of heart

RIGHT VENTRICLE

LEFT VENTRICLE

INFERIOR VENA CAVA

SEPTUM
Thick wall of muscle dividing heart

AORTA

What's a heart attack?

You have a far greater chance of dying of a heart attack than you have of getting run over by a bus. It's the most deadly killer we know, yet less than half of all men would recognise the symptoms of a heart attack and far fewer than that actually understand what one is.

If you're a man in the UK, you have a far greater chance of dying of a heart attack than if you lived in any other country. It's the cause of death for over 40,000 men in the UK each year. The really scary part is that most men are so undereducated about looking after their pumps that only around half of this number of deaths are unavoidable – because of hereditary factors, diabetes or naturally high blood pressure – the rest are a result of lifestyle choices. Remarkably, heart attacks are still one of the most misunderstood and frequently mistaken conditions.

A heart attack occurs when part of the heart's personal blood supply is cut off and the heart muscle tissue is deprived of oxygen. The most common cause of this is a blocked coronary artery, which can occur for two main reasons. The first is the long-term build-up of a hardened, fatty deposit called plaque on the artery's internal wall, caused

There may be trouble ahead

The warning signs of heart attack:

Breathlessness.

A crushing constriction of the chest, as if a band is being tightened around it.

Tightening of the shoulders and neck muscles.

Sweating.

Cold, pale, clammy skin.

Light-headedness or dizziness.

Nausea and maybe vomiting.

If you or somebody you are with suffers these symptoms, call an ambulance immediately. This is a serious medical condition and all you can do is attempt to make the sufferer as comfortable as possible until the professionals arrive.

Your resting heart rate should be between 60 and 100 beats per minute. Anything outside this for any prolonged amount of time and you should go to see your doctor.

by excess cholesterol (see page 128) in the blood, which eventually completely closes the tube. The other, far more common cause is that the surface of this plaque becomes rough or broken and causes a blood clot to form, which immediately blocks the artery. About 90 per cent of heart attacks are due to this latter cause.

As soon as the blockage happens, the heart's blood supply is interrupted, and the oxygen that the muscle walls need to keep beating is cut off with it. The muscle tissue immediately begins to deteriorate, and after roughly five minutes without oxygen the damage is irreversible and the tissue will die. Whether the heart can continue to function or not depends on the size of the blocked artery and how the rest of the heart can cope without it. In the cases of smaller blood vessels, neighbouring tubes take over

Britain still leads the world!

World Health Authority figures for the instances of heart attacks per 100,000 people:

United Kingdom	668
Finland	594
Poland	535
Lithuania	509
Czech Republic	508
Denmark	469
Russia	456
Belgium	399
Australia	398
New Zealand	393
Sweden	375
Iceland	370
USA	349
Germany	320
France	262
Italy	256
Switzerland	242
Hungary	150
China	86
Japan	80

and deliver extra blood to the area (though this is never healthy as it puts strain on the vessels). If the artery has been blocking up over time, often other arteries will have been expanding proportionately. Only if it is a big, major artery block will it shut the heart down straight away. Although it takes only five minutes for tissue to die, there can be more than two hours between the first warning signs and the actual heart attack, so it is vital not to ignore symptoms (see box, page 22). The best thing to do is to take one aspirin, as it limits the blood's tendency to clot by up to a third.

You are more likely to suffer a heart attack if ...

You have a family history of heart trouble

It is, to a degree, hereditary, and if both your parents suffered from coronary problems you are 40 per cent more likely to be at risk than somebody with no family history.

You have high blood pressure

Your heart has to continually work harder than it should do and is far more susceptible to damage.

Your cholesterol levels are high

This leads to a build-up of fatty deposits in your coronary arteries, restricting blood flow and making the arteries far more liable to blocking, as clots will form and bits of junk will break off the furred-up inner walls.

You are overweight

The obese are far more likely to experience serious heart trouble, as the heart has to beat so much harder to pump blood around the surplus poundage.

You are diabetic

You're at great risk. Roughly three-quarters of adult diabetics develop some sort of heart complaint.

You don't exercise

The heart is a muscle like any other, and if you don't keep working it out it will waste away. It will always work better if it is as strong as you can make it.

You are a heavy smoker

Smoking restricts the amount of oxygen available to the body and causes the heart to work so much harder that smokers have a 75 per cent chance of suffering a heart attack if they get over the age of 60.

You are more likely to survive a heart attack if ...

You take regular exercise

Regular exercise of other muscles in your body makes the heart work harder to supply the amount of oxygen needed in the blood. By beating harder and faster, the heart gets a good workout itself.

You avoid fatty foods

Watch out especially for cholesterol-loaded saturated fats and the death-in-a-bottle trans fats (see page 111) that are cropping up more and more in processed food. Even if you keep away from cholesterol you should avoid sugary stuff and other foods loaded with empty calories, as all they do is make you put on weight at the expense of proper nutrition.

You take half an aspirin a day

Aspirin, in small amounts, has been shown to thin the blood, which reduces the risk of heart attacks as your pump doesn't have to work so hard.

You incorporate certain foods in your diet

There are a number of foods that aren't merely not bad for your heart but will positively help it to function more efficiently. They're not at all boring either, as the list (see pages 48–50) includes cranberries, asparagus and salmon.

You give up smoking

Smoking is one of the biggest single contributors to heart disease in this country. The links are so apparent that within as little as 24 hours after stopping your chances of a heart attack drop massively.

Researchers in Switzerland have discovered that men are 60 per cent more likely to suffer a fatal heart attack during a televised sporting event. They advise keeping the blood flowing freely by getting up and moving about as much as possible while watching, and taking one aspirin beforehand – or you could support a team without a decent defence.

The circulatory system

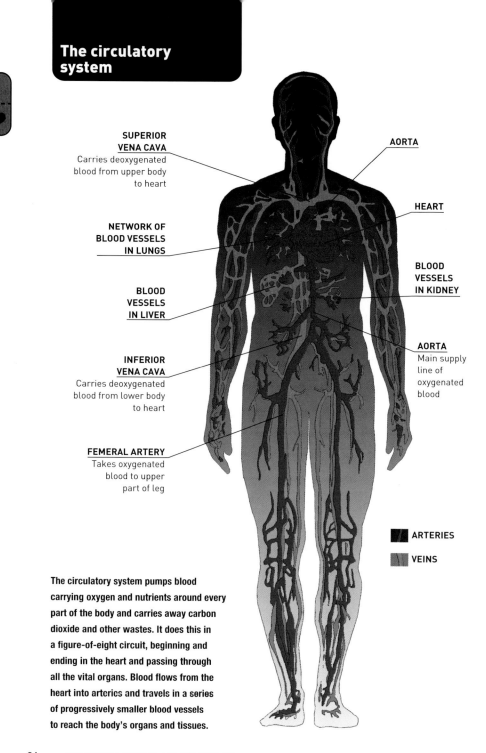

SUPERIOR VENA CAVA
Carries deoxygenated blood from upper body to heart

NETWORK OF BLOOD VESSELS IN LUNGS

BLOOD VESSELS IN LIVER

INFERIOR VENA CAVA
Carries deoxygenated blood from lower body to heart

FEMERAL ARTERY
Takes oxygenated blood to upper part of leg

AORTA

HEART

BLOOD VESSELS IN KIDNEY

AORTA
Main supply line of oxygenated blood

ARTERIES

VEINS

The circulatory system pumps blood carrying oxygen and nutrients around every part of the body and carries away carbon dioxide and other wastes. It does this in a figure-of-eight circuit, beginning and ending in the heart and passing through all the vital organs. Blood flows from the heart into arteries and travels in a series of progressively smaller blood vessels to reach the body's organs and tissues.

How the circulatory system works

Blood is, of course, the lifeblood of any man's body. If it's not moving then nothing gets done, which is why it's so important to understand how to keep the claret flowing.

As the heart beats, it pumps blood to every part of your body, delivering the oxygen the body needs to survive and the nutrients taken in as part of the food we eat. The oxygen-bearing blood exits the heart via the aorta, the largest blood vessel in the body, from where it flows into the body's main arteries (see illustration) and is distributed to the organs and tissues in a vast network of blood vessels of ever-decreasing sizes.

Blood simple

▌ **The average man has between 5 and** 6 litres (about 9 pints) of blood in his body. This is a little up on the traditional '8 pints' we were once estimated to have, because people have got bigger over the years.

▌ **The main ingredient of blood is a pale** yellow, watery fluid called plasma. Blood gets its colour from billions of red blood cells (corpuscles) suspended in the plasma.

▌ **There are roughly 500 times as many** red blood cells as there are white blood cells.

▌ **Veins appear blue when they show** through the skin because they are carrying oxygen-depleted blood, which is a darker red than oxygen-containing blood.

▌ **Most healthy men could lose** between 1 and 2 litres (1¾-3½ pint) of blood before bleeding becomes dangerous.

▌ **To seal a leaking wound, tiny blood** cells called platelets stick together to make a plug. Blood also produces a substance called fibrinogen that, when exposed to air, forms tiny adhesive fibres that ensnare the platelets, forming a clot and stopping the free flow of blood.

▌ **The average man has around 96,500** kilometres (60,000 miles) of blood vessels in his body. More than enough to go around the equator. Twice.

In case you were confused about this, the arteries take the blood away from the heart and carry it around your body to the outer regions. The blood is then returned to the heart by veins to begin the process all over again. Amazing piece of machinery, the human body.

Oxygen, glucose and other necessary nutrients are absorbed through the walls of the body's cells from the blood passing by in the capillaries. Each cell sops up precisely what it requires to keep it functioning, and once the blood has delivered this good stuff, it picks up the waste products. These are largely water and carbon dioxide – a by-product of the body's oxygen usage – which, together with other internally generated waste, are removed by the blood to various organs to be processed and expelled from the body. This happens as the blood makes its way back to the heart, travelling along a system of minuscule capillaries and then into a network of veins.

Although all blood flows through the heart (see page 21), not all blood flows through the entire layout of blood vessels.

There are a number of sub-circuits that carry out specific functions crucial to keeping the body working. The most important is the respiratory circulation, which carries deoxygenated blood from the heart, passes it through the lungs to be re-enriched with oxygen and returns it to the heart to be pumped around the body. Blood that flows through the stomach and intestines then passes through the liver, where nutrients picked up from the digestive tract are processed before being delivered to the heart to be pumped around the whole system.

Of the waste products collected, carbon dioxide is delivered back to the lungs where it can be expelled in exhaled breath, while waste from food is returned to the liver and kidneys and processed for excretion.

It's in the blood

Healthy blood is as important as a healthy circulatory system. Here are a brace of blood disorders you ought to know about.

ANAEMIA

The most common blood disorder, this is a deficiency in red blood cells that vastly reduces the amount of oxygen delivered around the body. The result is fatigue, mental tiredness and a paler skin. Anaemia is usually the result of an iron deficiency, which can be overcome by eating plenty of leafy green vegetables or liver, or taking an iron supplement.

SICKLE CELL DISEASE

This disorder, often called sickle cell anaemia, is so called because the red blood cells become an abnormal sickle shape. These deformed cells are too brittle to get through the tiny capillaries and deliver oxygen to the tissues, and they cause blockages by preventing normal blood flow. The symptoms include fatigue, breathlessness and sometimes severe bone pain. Sickle cell disease is genetic and will be inherited if both parents have the defective gene – which doesn't necessarily mean they have the condition; they may just be carriers. The condition is far more prevalent in people of African-Caribbean and Asian origin – one in ten is believed to have the defective gene – so if you are of that genetic group you are advised to investigate your family medical history before starting a family of your own. Sickle cell disease causes recurring bouts of illness throughout life and cannot be cured. Anyone affected should avoid over-exertion that demands a great deal of oxygen. Folic acid supplements can aid the production of healthy red blood cells.

Feel the pressure

High blood pressure affects one in five men! It can attack your heart! It can kill without warning! It is one of the biggest men's health issues and is ignored at your peril.

Dangerously high blood pressure, or hypertension, has no advance guard, it has no symptoms and can affect even the healthiest-feeling men, so it's vital that you are aware of its potential menace from your mid-thirties onwards. In other words, get your blood pressure tested before your blood pressure tests you.

To do the test, your doctor inflates a restrictive cuff around your arm to stop blood flow. Then, as the cuff is deflated, the pressure of the released blood is measured on a meter. The readings are made up of two numbers – 140/80, for instance. The higher number, known as systolic pressure, represents blood pressure as the heart muscle contracts and the lower number, known as diastolic pressure, is the reading taken as the heart muscle relaxes. Typical readings for a healthy 40-year-old would be 130/80, with a younger man having considerably lower than that, say, 120/68, or a 50-year-old being closer to 150/85.

Check the pressure regularly

Roughly one in five British men has high blood pressure, but far fewer than that are actually aware of it. Every man should have his blood pressure checked, and checks ought to increase in frequency as the years roll by. Get it done once in your twenties, and, provided nothing is wrong, every three years throughout your thirties, every two years throughout your forties and annually after that.

Don't settle for just one check, as that might not necessarily give a true picture of your blood pressure. Ask for several tests over the course of a month and your doctor will much better be able to work out your condition from them.

Window-rattling snoring can cause blood pressure to rise while you are asleep. It means that the amount of oxygen you are taking in is reduced, so blood pressure rises as the heart works harder to service the body with what oxygen is available.

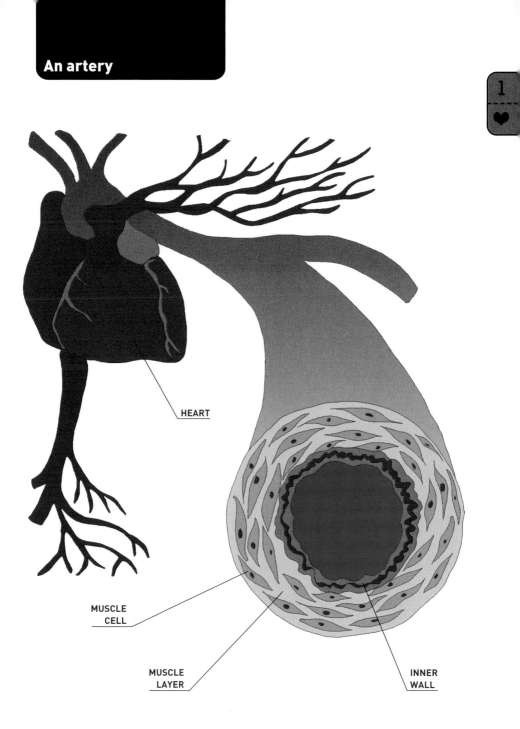

HEART

MUSCLE
CELL

MUSCLE
LAYER

INNER
WALL

Vigorous exercise – or vigorous sex – might cause blood pressure to rise, but this will only be temporary and should not affect you long term. Also, there is no reason why a man with high blood pressure shouldn't lead a full and active sex life, provided he looks after his circulatory system as much as possible and knows what his limits are. If you are worried, talk to your doctor and be prepared to be imaginative.

There is no such thing as normal blood pressure across the board. Everybody's is different and may vary quite a lot during the average day. Blood pressure is lowest while you are asleep and highest after physical activity, and during a normal day usually peaks about five hours after you get up. To get an accurate measure of your blood pressure, the test should be the result of several different readings taken over a number of days. But while the systolic reading tends to go up with age by roughly ten points per decade, from around 120 for a 20-year-old, the diastolic reading is more of a constant. Hence doctors tend to pay more attention to it and any reading over 90 is cause for concern.

High blood pressure can be inherited, so it's worth looking into your family's medical history, but increasingly these days it is caused by outside elements. One of the biggest causes of high blood pressure is stress, which can cause the heart to beat faster; obesity is another major hypertension contributor as the heart has to work so much harder to pump blood around your body. A high cholesterol level won't help either, as it furs up the arteries, making the heart push harder. Smoking has much the same effect, as the blood of a heavy smoker becomes considerably thicker than normal.

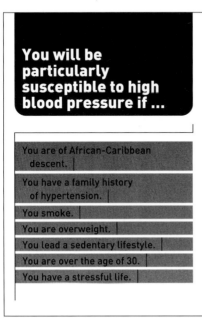

You will be particularly susceptible to high blood pressure if ...

You are of African-Caribbean descent.

You have a family history of hypertension.

You smoke.

You are overweight.

You lead a sedentary lifestyle.

You are over the age of 30.

You have a stressful life.

Pressure drop

Virtually any man over the age of 40 is potentially at risk from hypertension, and certain of those among us have a greater chance than others. However, there are precautions we can all take to make sure the doctor's gauges don't go up further than they have to.

CUT DOWN ON SALT

Recent surveys show that the countries with the most salt in their diets are the countries with the highest levels of hypertension – the USA in particular, but we are not far behind.

The reason for this is that excess salt in your system means excess water – salt attracts water – and if your kidneys cannot expel it then blood volume increases, raising the pressure. As well as simply not shaking so much salt on to your meals, avoid processed food (which is nearly always overly rich in salt), salty snacks, cured meat or fish and stock cubes.

EAT MORE OILY FISH

Unfortunately, people in the West eat a disproportionately small amount of fish. If we

Hey! Lard ass! Put that cigarette out!

There are no two ways about it: the two biggest causes of high blood pressure are being overweight and smoking. It won't matter how many other precautions you take if you can admit to one or both of these – you are a prime candidate for hypertension. The reasons are really rather obvious.

Smoking reduces the amount of oxygen you take in and therefore the heart needs to work harder to pump what it does get around the system; plus smokers' blood is notably thicker than non-smokers' (see pages 52–67). As if that wasn't enough, your blood vessels are likely to be narrower as

smoking encourages a build-up of harmful cholesterol that can clog up your pipes (see Cholesterol Explained, page 128).

Being fat is just as dangerous. Quite apart from the chances that what you eat is increasing your cholesterol levels, every extra kilo of fat you carry means that your blood has a greater distance to travel around your body. This puts a much greater strain on your heart, and your blood pressure will rise accordingly. Lose that unsightly belly and your blood pressure will fall by four or five points.

raised that level to, say, two meals with fish a week, we would be considerably reducing the risks of hypertension. Oily fish, particularly salmon and mackerel, have a high concentrate of the fatty acid omega-3, which helps combat excess cholesterol levels and also thins the blood, allowing it to flow more easily around a less-than-perfect system.

INCREASE YOUR CALCIUM INTAKE

Because many men worry about the cholesterol content of dairy products, they cut out milk, cheese and butter, and so sacrifice a useful source of calcium. Recent research shows that men with even relatively mild calcium deficiencies have a much greater likelihood of having high blood pressure too. So either take a calcium supplement or get back on the dairy. Just make sure it's the non-fat variety.

WATCH THOSE STRESS LEVELS

High-stress situations can cause blood pressure to spike, and a perpetually stressful situation – business problems or a bad marriage, for instance – can lead to continuing hypertension. If it is impossible to avoid the causes of the stress, then calm yourself down with relaxation techniques such as yoga, meditation or tai chi (see pages 176–181).

GET SOME EXERCISE

Not only will exercise help you to lose weight (see pages 46–47) and build muscle, but a continuous programme of aerobic exercise – such as running, swimming, cycling or playing sports – has other long-term benefits. Exercises like these increase your cardiovascular efficiency, meaning that your heart and lungs will work better and your circulation and its oxygen-carrying capacity will improve.

CUT BACK ON THE BOOZE

There is a definite link between drinking too much and hypertension. Excess alcohol over a long period of time can prove positively dangerous for those who already have raised blood pressure. Men with high blood pressure should cut back to no more than 14 units a week (21 is the recommended maximum) and those with normal blood pressure should think about doing the same.

TRY DANDELIONS

The French eat them all the time as a salad leaf, and the percentage of French men with high blood pressure is considerably smaller than in the UK – but then that could be all the red wine and garlic (see page 49)! Dandelion leaves are delicious and can help to lower harmful cholesterol levels and reduce blood pressure because they thin the blood.

Circulation breakdown

There are several more very good reasons why you should keep your blood lines open.

ATHEROSCLEROSIS

This is a furring-up and thickening of the arteries that gets worse with age, restricting the free flow of blood and increasing the likelihood of internal blockages. Atherosclerosis arises when excess cholesterol carried in the bloodstream begins to stick to the lining of the arteries. Over time these fatty deposits, called plaques, build up, decreasing the internal diameter of the blood vessels (think of water pipes getting furred up inside with an accumulation of limescale).

Eventually, the artery walls themselves become thickened, making the passageway even narrower. Atherosclerosis can lead to serious and possibly fatal diseases such as heart attacks and strokes.

Prevent it by not smoking, watching your weight and cutting back on foods containing harmful fats (see pages 126–31).

VARICOSE VEINS

Those blue, knotted leg veins are not simply a worry for old ladies who probably wear headscarves in the house. Around one per cent of all adult men have been to their

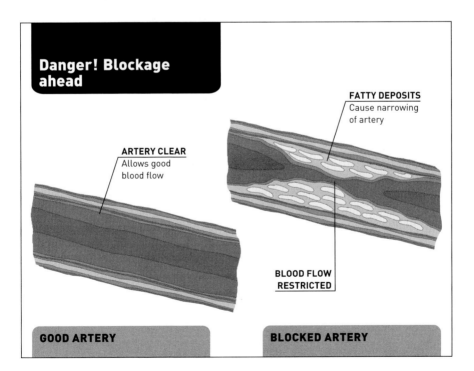

Danger! Blockage ahead

FATTY DEPOSITS
Cause narrowing of artery

ARTERY CLEAR
Allows good blood flow

BLOOD FLOW RESTRICTED

GOOD ARTERY

BLOCKED ARTERY

doctor with concerns about varicose veins. They can be a genuine worry for anybody who is on his feet for most of the time, more so if that doesn't involve much walking about. Varicose veins are caused by weakness of the one-way valves in the leg veins, which allows blood to seep backwards and pool in the superficial blood vessels just beneath the skin. These vessels become swollen and look blue because they contain deoxygenated blood. The legs may ache and sometimes the skin over the veins becomes itchy. Varicose veins can occur elsewhere in the body, such as around the anus when they are known as haemorrhoids, but are most common in the legs because once the valves have jammed, gravity makes sure the blood descends.

Prevent them by moving about as much as possible if you have to keep on your feet all day, and avoid crossing your ankles when you sit down. Put your feet up (above your waist) whenever possible, and don't smoke as it increases the toxins in the blood that won't be cleared from the affected areas.

STROKE

Although fewer than two in every 1000 people in the UK suffer from a stroke, and the majority of them are over 65 years old, the dangers shouldn't be dismissed. A stroke happens when the blood supply to part of the brain is cut off and those particular brain cells can't get any oxygen. The results of a stroke, which can include weakness or numbness on one side of the body, slurred speech and blurred vision, depend on what part of the brain is affected. There are two main causes: a blood clot in one of the arteries of the brain (cerebral thrombosis); or a rupturing of one of the brain's blood vessels (cerebral haemorrhage).

Prevent it by keeping your circulatory system as healthy as possible (as discussed above) and taking half an aspirin a day to thin the blood.

BLOOD CLOTS

Although the blood is designed to clot on exposure to the air and thus seal cuts and wounds, internal clotting (thrombosis) can cause all sorts of problems by blocking blood vessels. Clots can be caused by an enzyme imbalance that reduces the blood's anticoagulating capabilities, or they can form around fatty deposits on artery linings (see Atherosclerosis, page 35). Blood clots are more likely to form in a slow-moving circulatory system and can eventually break off and float around the bloodstream with the potential to cause serious damage.

Prevent them by keeping your cholesterol level down and taking all precautions to keep your blood flowing swiftly.

Deep vein thrombosis (DVT)

DVT deserves to be taken seriously. It occurs when a blood clot forms in one of the larger veins deep inside the legs (hence the name) where any potential clot can be a lot bigger than one formed in smaller veins nearer the surface. While the clot may not cause any damage where it is, relatively large chunks can break off and travel to the veins that service the heart and lungs, causing dangerous blockage. Long-haul fliers are susceptible to DVT because cramped conditions force them to remain more or less motionless for long periods of time, constricting blood flow in the legs and encouraging clotting. Serious effects may not occur until after the flight, when the person is moving about again and blood starts flowing freely, possibly carrying the clot through the system.

PREVENT IT BY

Getting up and walking about as much as your fellow travellers can stand, or rotating and flexing your ankles. Try to extend your knees every half hour.

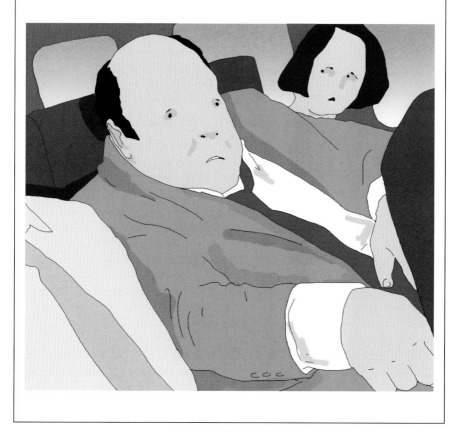

Your achy breaky heart

Avoid the clogged arteries and the potential blood clots and you still might not be out of the woods.

ANGINA

Angina is a strangling pain that seems to constrict your chest and can extend to the shoulders, neck and jaw. It is brought about by a poor supply of oxygenated blood to the heart muscles, often because of narrowed arteries. The pain is most commonly triggered by some heavy-duty physical exertion that puts an extra strain on the heart. As the heart pumps harder so it needs more oxygen, and if an adequate supply isn't forthcoming the heart muscles suffer cramps. Angina attacks can last up to 20 minutes and are more likely to occur after a heavy meal or in cold conditions. Anybody with a poorly functioning circulatory system will be far more susceptible to angina, and attacks are usually taken as early warning signs of more serious heart trouble in the future.

ARRHYTHMIAS

Your resting heart rate should be somewhere between 60 and 100 beats per minute. Anything either faster or slower than this, or a heartbeat that follows an irregular rhythm, is known as an arrhythmia. An abnormal heart rate is usually a warning that something is wrong either in the heart itself or elsewhere in the body: the heart's internal pacemaker (the sinoatrial node) may be

How dangerous is sex?

Provided you're not doing it with your neighbour's wife and he's a karate black belt, sex needn't be dangerous at all for anybody with a dodgy heart. The rules are pretty much the same as for anybody with high blood pressure (see page 30) as the increased heart rate during sex – even merely to maintain an erection – puts added strain on your pump. Together with your partner, explore possibilities you might not have considered before, acts that involve less exertion on your part, and even consider ways of pleasuring your partner without actual intercourse. It is important to let your partner know how you are feeling about this, and it can serve to bring you closer together. However, if you have serious concerns or a very bad heart, speak to your doctor before making any decisions. If having sex causes angina attacks or other chest pains, stop immediately.

malfunctioning; the thyroid gland is not working properly; there are heart valve problems or coronary artery disease; or there is a hormone imbalance within the body. Symptoms of arrhythmia include palpitations, dizziness, breathlessness, fainting and chest pains. If you experience any or all of these you should see your doctor as soon as possible. Most arrhythmias do not require treatment, although in more serious cases drugs such as beta blockers may be used or an artificial pacemaker may be fitted.

ARTERY SPASM

This is an unexplained and, thankfully, relatively uncommon condition when a section of the coronary artery walls contracts and cuts off the blood flow for as long as the spasm lasts. Spasms are as likely to occur in healthy arteries as they are in clogged pipes.

CONGESTIVE HEART FAILURE

This is exactly what it sounds like, and occurs when the heart weakens and cannot pump blood out through the arteries as fast

Medicine

Your doctor may write a prescription to combat your heart condition. These are the three drugs most likely to be involved:

BETA BLOCKERS

These reduce blood pressure by lowering the resting heart rate, and restrict the degree the rate rises during exercise by blocking the production of hormones in the body that produce the increase. Side effects of beta blockers include those associated with a too low pulse, such as fatigue and erectile dysfunction.

NITRATE-BASED DRUGS

Used to treat angina, these drugs expand the blood vessels and so improve blood flow. Their effect is more or less instant and they can relieve the pain while an angina attack is happening. Nitrate drugs can also be taken to prevent angina occurring but excessive use – some angina sufferers take them on a daily basis – can be counter-productive, as the body develops a tolerance to them.

ANTI-CLOTTING DRUGS

Just as the name implies, these restrict the blood's ability to clot. They work by reducing the production or activity of the enzymes needed to form blood clots. The most commonly prescribed anti-clotting drugs are hepanin, which is injected, and phenindione and warfarin, which are both taken orally. There is also aspirin, which is known for its anti-clotting and blood-thinning properties.

Testing, one two, testing

If you go to see the doctor with suspected heart problems, a number of tests can be carried out that take the science of heart examination way beyond simply listening through a stethoscope. It will help your case greatly to be aware of what is on offer.

CHEST X-RAY

This is the most simple form of electronic examination. A straight-forward chest X-ray usually reveals enough to tell a doctor if there is any abnormality regarding the size and shape of your heart, if there is a blockage in the valves or arteries and if there has been any build-up of blood or fluid in the chambers or connecting passages.

ELECTROCARDIOGRAPHY (ECG)

An ECG machine measures the electrical impulses that occur in a heart immediately before the contraction of the muscle and the heartbeat. It records any irregularities of the heartbeat that might indicate muscle disorder and, by showing up any variations in a normal pattern, can point out potential coronary artery disease or blockage.

ECHOCARDIOGRAPHY

This records ultrasound images of the heart – simply put, it creates pictures drawn from a complex series of sounds being sent out and returned, not unlike a marine depth-finder. Echocardiography is particularly useful in finding structural defects of the heart walls, valves and arteries, and can detect abnormalities in valve function as it shows the valve flaps opening and closing.

ANGIOGRAPHY

A contrasting fluid is injected into the heart's circulatory system through a catheter inserted in the groin (see page 45) and a quick succession of X-rays are taken showing how the dye is moving through the system – producing something like a rudimentary movie. By showing the internal flow in this manner, angiography gives a vivid picture of the state of the arteries and allows a doctor to decide if further action for blocked or narrowing blood vessels needs to be taken.

CT (COMPUTED TOMOGRAPHY) SCANNING

You will be rolled into a full body scanner, where X-rays are passed through the body at varying angles, presenting a series of computer-generated cross-section images of any part of your body and what is going on inside it. The technique is particularly useful in heart examination, as the images are incredibly detailed and reveal even the smallest abnormalities of the arteries, valves or heart walls.

as it enters through the veins. As a result, the right-side chambers overfill with blood and eventually either the surplus blood ends up in the lungs or the heart stops. Congestive heart failure can come about through aging or following prolonged inactivity – such as a period of convalescence.

VALVE DISORDERS

The heart has four valves that control the one-way flow of blood through the heart chambers. Any valve malfunction can be serious and may need to be corrected by surgery. Often, heart valve problems are congenital (present from birth), but they can develop as a person ages – the valves literally wear out – or as the result of reduced blood supply through the heart brought on by circulatory disorders.

The most common problem is a leaky valve, when the flaps (cusps) that make up a valve fail to close properly and allow a backwash of blood into the chamber it is supposed to be leaving. As a result, the first chamber dangerously overfills and

eventually the heart will stop. Valve prolapse is progressive, and can be heard by a doctor as an abnormal heart sound, or 'murmur'. Another disorder, called stenosis, is the narrowing and possible eventual closure of a valve that is usually due to a build-up of calcium deposits, particularly in older people. Bacterial endocarditis is an infection of the valves, which can cause complications in valve prolapse or, if untreated, become a serious problem in itself. This disorder is not very common, though, and has its highest instances among intravenous drug users.

Serious valve disorders may require surgery and, although some conditions can be corrected under the knife a valve transplant is the most likely option. A malfunctioning valve will be removed and replaced with one from a human donor, a synthetic manufactured unit or possibly tissue from a pig's heart, which is approximately the same size as a man's.

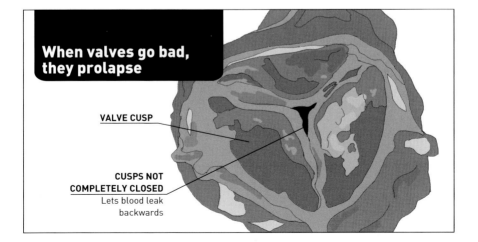

When valves go bad, they prolapse

VALVE CUSP

CUSPS NOT
COMPLETELY CLOSED
Lets blood leak
backwards

Heart surgery for beginners

When dietary changes, medication or an exercise routine aren't enough to keep your arteries open and your heart pumping, the only option left is surgery. When a major blockage has been sudden and unannounced – a massive heart attack – and has to be shifted equally quickly, you'll most likely wake up in the recovery room having had your chest opened and closed again.

Although heart surgery isn't exactly to be recommended, it isn't nearly as risky as you might suppose and even comes with a number of different options for getting your tubes clear again.

CORONARY ARTERY BYPASS

This is exactly what it says on the tin: the operation creates a bypass around a blocked coronary artery by grafting on a length of healthy artery or vein to carry the blood past the obstruction. Veins used in bypass surgery are usually taken from the patient's leg, while arteries are most likely to be taken from somewhere else within the chest. A bypass is the most commonly performed operation for treating atherosclerosis (see page 35), as transplanted arteries seldom fur up again. These operations have been carried out all over the world since the end of the 1960s. You may hear the terms 'double' and 'triple' bypass surgery – these refer to the number of coronary arteries that have had bypasses grafted on to them.

BALLOON ANGIOPLASTY

First used at the end of the 1970s, this technique is used to widen coronary arteries that are narrowed or blocked by fatty deposits. Balloon angioplasty has something of the Fantastic Voyage about it, as it is a closed rather than an open heart procedure. A catheter (a very thin, very flexible tube) with a tiny balloon attached to the end of it is inserted into the femoral artery in the top of the patient's thigh with the aid of a flexible guide wire. This is then pushed up into the affected coronary artery (see illustrations, pages 44 and 45). Once inside the narrowed area, the balloon is inflated and deflated a number of times, getting slightly larger each time and being held fully inflated for several seconds. The expanding balloon both compresses the fatty deposit and pushes the artery wall outwards. This opens up the artery and allows the blood to flow freely once more. The balloon is then withdrawn. Although angioplasty is nearly always successful there is a high percentage of repeat procedures as narrowed arteries have a tendency to close up again.

Coronary artery bypass

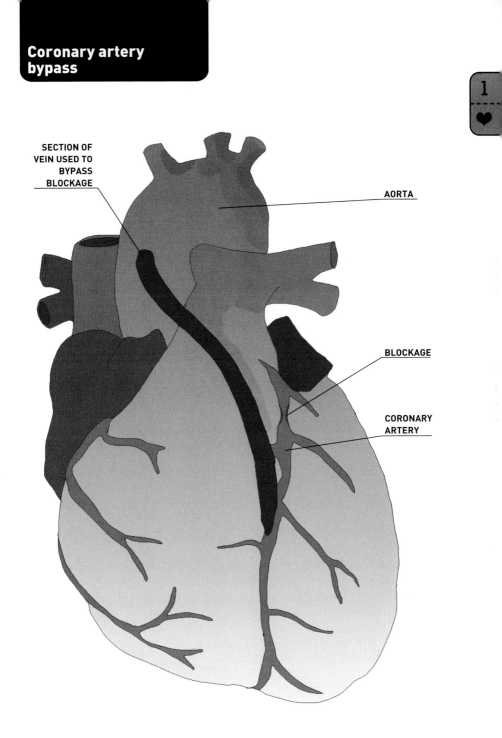

SECTION OF VEIN USED TO BYPASS BLOCKAGE

AORTA

BLOCKAGE

CORONARY ARTERY

STENT INSERTION

This relatively recently developed procedure takes angioplasty one stage further and has a much higher permanent success rate. After the angioplasty procedure has been performed a plastic mesh support, the stent, is inserted into the artery to prevent it closing again.

HEART TRANSPLANT

Pretty self-explanatory: this involves taking your malfunctioning old heart out and putting one that works properly back in its place. Yes, it can be done. No, you don't ever want to be in the situation where it is even being thought about as an option.

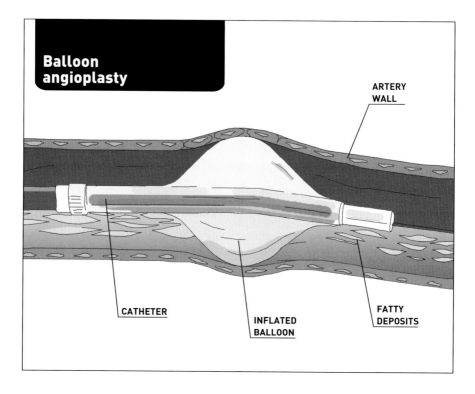

Balloon angioplasty

ARTERY WALL

CATHETER

INFLATED BALLOON

FATTY DEPOSITS

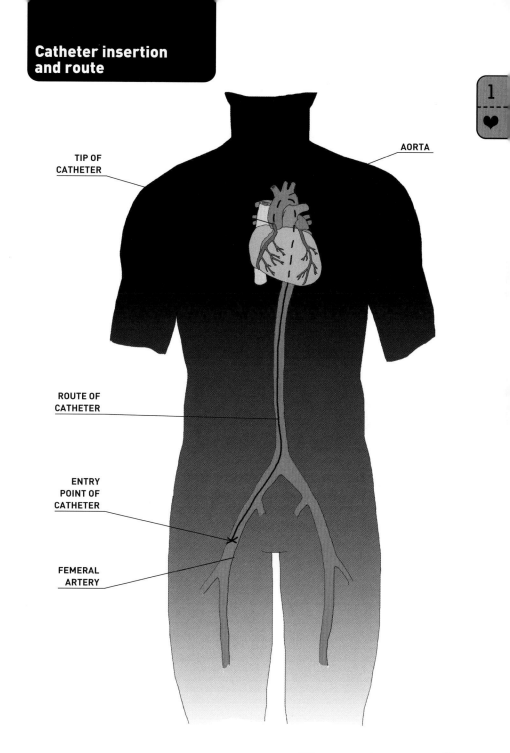

Catheter insertion and route

TIP OF CATHETER

AORTA

ROUTE OF CATHETER

ENTRY POINT OF CATHETER

FEMERAL ARTERY

How exercise can help your heart

If you're concerned about your heart – and you ought to be – then you should be looking at taking some sort of regular exercise. At best, it could save your life; at least, it will simply make you feel better.

Exercise can combat heart disease because a man's heart is really just a big muscle and as such needs to be worked out to keep it strong and pumping. A stronger heart is automatically a healthier heart. Think of it as you might a powerful car engine: idling while you're sitting, but when called on to accelerate – when you get physically

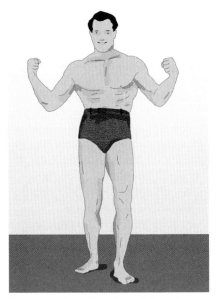

Would you kick sand in this man's face? You, too, can look like this if only you'd exercise more.

The best exercise routine is the one you'll stick to

Don't be over-ambitious and try for a programme that will either be too much for you to complete or may even do you physical damage. Start off with something that stretches you but won't put you off, and that you have the time and facilities to keep up with. Don't choose a gym-based programme if you're unlikely to go to the gym regularly; and make sure your programme doesn't take an impractical amount of time – 'I'm too busy to work out today!' is probably the hardest working excuse in the book.

active – it revs a bit quicker but is never putting itself under any strain. Then, if the driver puts his foot down briefly, or you have to do something very strenuous, it's still well within its capabilities.

The idea is to be able to cope with normal circulatory circumstances without thinking about them, then to have power in reserve to deal with any of the possible malfunctions we've looked at in this section. The way to supercharge your pump is to work out other muscles in the body in a series of aerobic exercises.

'Aerobic' means dependent on oxygen, and an aerobic exercise is one that requires the supply of oxygen being delivered through

Any exercise is better than none at all

But that doesn't mean the arduous trek from the sofa to the fridge and back again is going to be enough to keep your heart healthy. Start with a simple – and simply obvious – exercise routine: get off the train or bus a stop earlier and walk the rest of the way; take the stairs instead of the lift; use a washroom on a different floor from your workstation; run up the stairs at home instead of walking; add an extra few streets on to the dog's walk, and so on. A good way to start getting fit is to look for ways to incorporate exercise into your daily routine.

Your capacity for aerobic exercise will increase rapidly once you start and what may have begun as one 15-minute session per day will soon turn into a longer period or more than one shorter workout. Running, cycling, skipping, swimming, stair-climbing, power walking or rowing are all ideal aerobic exercises. The optimum time for a session is half an hour, plus five minutes on either side for warming up and warming down.

When exercising aerobically, check your heart rate frequently. You are aiming for a heartbeat that is between 50 and 80 per cent of the maximum for your age. Calculate what this should be by subtracting your age from 220: thus, a man of 35 will have a maximum heart rate of 185. Fifty per cent of that is 92.5 and 80 per cent is 148; so during aerobic exercise a man should be aiming to sustain a heart rate of somewhere between those two figures. (For a more detailed look at exercising for health, see pages 132–39.)

the bloodstream to increase and remain increased for at least fifteen minutes. This is achieved through continuous, prolonged working out, keeping the muscles demanding additional oxygen. In order for the bloodstream to deliver this extra oxygen the heart has to pump harder. If aerobic workouts are carried out over a period of time, the heart grows in size and capability, in exactly the same way as any other regularly exercised muscle would.
A useful by-product of aerobic exercise is that this sort of sustained workout requires enormous calorie burning to fuel the exertions, therefore any excess weight you are carrying should start to fall off.

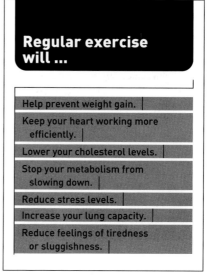

Regular exercise will ...

Help prevent weight gain.

Keep your heart working more efficiently.

Lower your cholesterol levels.

Stop your metabolism from slowing down.

Reduce stress levels.

Increase your lung capacity.

Reduce feelings of tiredness or sluggishness.

Twenty foods your heart would like you to eat

While exercise is vital to maintaining a happy, healthy heart, so is what you eat. Luckily, this doesn't mean a diet of lentils and brown rice – although that wouldn't do you any harm – as many of the foods that are best for your heart and blood pressure are some of the most interesting you'll find on any menu.

ALMONDS

Like so many nuts, these are a good source of protein. As a bonus, almonds contain circulation-boosting fibre and vitamin E, which helps to combat heart disease.

APPLE JUICE

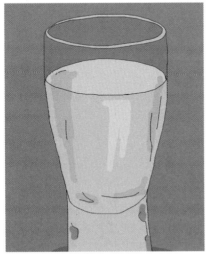

The natural antioxidants in apple juice drastically slow down the effects of harmful cholesterol in the bloodstream.

ASPARAGUS

This is rich in folic acid, a vitamin that helps to prevent narrowing of the blood vessels in the legs (which is a particular risk to smokers).

BANANAS

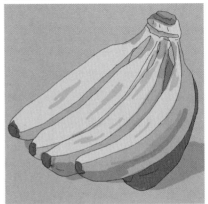

The yellow fruit is a rich source of potassium, which is essential for maintaining a regular cardiac rhythm.

BLACK PEPPER

Black pepper purifies the blood by filtering out a large amount of potential toxins.

BLUEBERRIES

Rich in antioxidants, reliable blood thinners and cholesterol blasters, blueberries should be a vital part of your diet.

BREAKFAST

A healthy breakfast, that is. American research has shown that people who eat breakfast are almost 50 per cent less likely to suffer heart attacks than those who skip it. The reason? It keeps their metabolism working far more efficiently and therefore able to cope with food during the rest of the day with relative ease.

CRANBERRIES

Research at the University of Massachusetts has revealed that cranberries guard against the effects of a stroke. A daily serving of the berries provided enough protection to keep brain cells from dying during a simulated stroke.

GARLIC

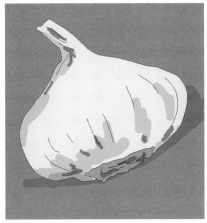

The words 'too', 'much' and 'garlic' are contradictions in terms and should never be seen in the same sentence. Garlic doesn't just ward off vampires, it wards off practically everything else that could do you harm. The magic bulb protects your pump by lowering artery-clogging cholesterol levels (see page 128), and reduces your blood

pressure by thinning the blood. Shame something so good for your heart can be so bad for your love life – best get your partner to eat as much of it as you do.

MARGARINE

This can be a valuable source of polyunsaturated fat, which lowers cholesterol levels across the board. Check the label, though, as brands vary.

OLIVE OIL

A monounsaturated fat that is much kinder to your heart than dairy fats, as it works to lower harmful cholesterol. It's still a fat, though, so treat it with respect.

RED CHILLI PEPPERS

These thin the blood to keep circulation moving and reduce cholesterol levels.

RED WINE

One glass a day can be a valuable source of chromium, a mineral that works to regulate cholesterol levels in the bloodstream.

ROOT GINGER

More than just a traditional stomach medicine, root ginger has a powerful effect on the circulatory system, reducing the likelihood of blood clots and keeping the blood flowing easily by reducing any stickiness.

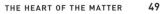

SALMON

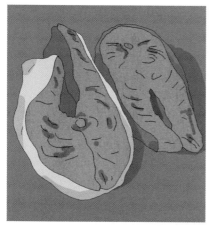

All oily fish – including mackerel or sardines, for instance – is rich in the essential fatty acid omega-3, which gives protection against heart disease and raises your circulatory efficiency by thinning the blood, but salmon has more of it than the others.

SKINLESS CHICKEN

Chicken breasts are a useful source of protein; however, there is a layer of artery-endangering fat just below the skin. Lose the skin, lose the fat.

SPINACH

A bit of a superstar, spinach is incredibly rich in iron, which is needed for the production of red blood cells and the prevention of anaemia. This veg is also a vital source of folic acid, a vitamin that works hard to keep your blood free-flowing.

TEA

Green or black, regular tea drinking – which means several cups a day – cuts cholesterol by up to 15 per cent.

WHOLE GRAINS

A very good source of insoluble fibre, whole grains can actually help you cut down on overeating. They need to be chewed for a long time and as the action of chewing triggers sensors in the brain that tell you your stomach is full, whole grains fool you into thinking you have had more to eat than is the case.

YOGHURT

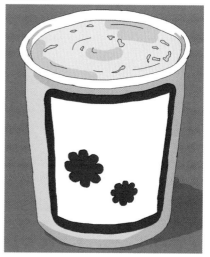

This is a good source of calcium, and calcium intake is inversely proportioned to blood pressure – the lower the calcium consumption, the higher the blood pressure. Also, if you are looking to lose weight, calcium helps you to burn fat faster and inhibits the amount you'll put back on.

What not to eat

BUTTER AND FULL FAT DAIRY PRODUCTS

All full fat dairy foods are rich in saturated fats, which increase the levels of harmful cholesterol and do your arteries no good at all. Avoid butter by using a substitute containing monounsaturated fat (olive oil spread) or polyunsaturated fat (sunflower oil spread) and switch to non-fat cheese and milk.

SALT

The regular amount of salt most of us sprinkle on our food is fine, but too much is bad for the heart because it increases the volume of blood and so raises your blood pressure – just as if you put too much oil in your car. People of African-Caribbean descent are far more likely to be affected by excess salt than those of the Caucasian persuasion – as many as three-quarters of all black people are 'salt sensitive'. Asians also tend to have too much salt in their diet.

LOADS OF BOOZE

Whereas drinking in moderation – especially red wine – is proven to have a beneficial effect on the heart, sinking a skinful on a regular basis can be very dangerous. Alcohol weakens the action of the heart muscle, so to compensate the heart speeds up, raising blood pressure. Continued heavy drinking produces a build-up of fat in the liver, which then cannot process toxins out of the blood with its usual efficiency; in turn, this impairs the blood's ability to deliver oxygen to the body's tissues. The heart then has to work even harder.

COFFEE

If drunk in moderation by reasonably healthy people, coffee is of no danger whatsoever. In fact, the pulse-quickening jolt from a decent caffeine shot is what most of us need to get going in the morning. In providing this lift, though, caffeine causes the heart to pump faster by a couple of beats per minute, raising blood pressure by up to five points. After one cup of coffee, the heart rate falls back to normal pretty soon, but constant caffeine hits throughout the day keep the rate – and blood pressure – raised for too long to be entirely safe. As caffeine tolerance is easily acquired – people tend to drink more and more to get the same invigorating experience – and blood pressure can soon creep into the danger levels. Anybody with existing high blood pressure should be very careful about caffeine intake. It's not only coffee that contains high caffeine levels, of course. There are high levels in fizzy soft drinks and tea.

The truth about smoking

It might have been big and it might even have been clever when you were eleven. Nowadays, though, you wheeze when you run for a train, your skin looks like parchment and a transatlantic flight leaves you in bits. Isn't it time you faced the facts?

It would be pointless to tell you smoking isn't good for you – if you had the intelligence in the first place to pick this book up and read it, then you're bright enough to know smoking is bad. Precisely how bad, however, is something you might not quite have come to terms with.

Sure, we all know about lung cancer, which has been directly linked to smoking due to the high levels of carcinogens (cancer-causing substances) in cigarette smoke, but these same carcinogens can also cause cancer in the stomach, throat, mouth, kidneys and pancreas. Smoking is one of the most frequent causes of heart disease, as the effects of tobacco put enormous strain on

A word to the wise

Three hundred deaths a day in Great Britain are directly attributed to smoking.

Over 25,000 men are diagnosed with lung cancer every year.

Every year smoking kills six times as many people as traffic accidents, poisoning, murder, manslaughter, suicide and HIV combined.

Ninety per cent of all lung cancer cases are smoking related, as are 30 per cent of all other cancers.

A quarter of all cot deaths occur in households where there is one or more heavy smokers.

A 20-a-day smoker is three times more likely than a non-smoker to develop heart disease – this increases proportionately to the number of cigarettes smoked.

Although smoking is declining among older men (40-plus), it is on the rise among the under thirties. The younger you start, the more cumulative damage you will do and the less likely you are to quit.

'Smoking' is now acceptable as the cause of death on a death certificate.

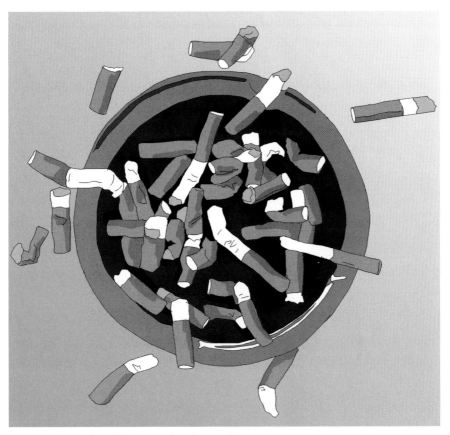

If this is your idea of breakfast, you are in serious trouble.

the circulatory system: reducing the amount of oxygen in the bloodstream, raising levels of dangerous cholesterol, increasing the likelihood of blood clots and thickening the blood to slow down its flow. This last point has particular implications, as it leads to disorders such as ischaemia (poor blood supply) in the legs, which causes pain when walking, and damages blood vessels in the brain, increasing the chances of a stroke.

Then there's the fact that the smoke greatly reduces the efficiency of the tiny fibres that line your airways and act as filters to keep debris out of the lungs. Once these aren't working properly all manner of foreign bodies get into the lungs. Lasting lung damage takes place as the crap starts to build up, leaving you short of breath and far more susceptible to coughs, colds and lung infections in general.

Because the connection between smoking and killer diseases such as heart attacks and cancer (only about eight per cent of men survive lung cancer) is so clear cut,

What cigarettes do for you – the top ten

Apart from, obviously, burning your money, making your clothes smell and sending you to huddle in doorways like some sort of well-tailored bum, cigarettes also:

1 Give you a variety of cancers

Smoking is the highest cause of lung cancer on the planet and is the major contributing factor to cancers of the mouth, throat, kidneys and pancreas.

2 Shorten your life

Less than ten per cent of all lung cancer patients survive.

3 Poison you

Smoking introduces a range of poisons including arsenic, formaldehyde, hydrogen cyanide and lead into your system.

4 Cause erectile dysfunction

In terms of duration and rigidity, and even if you can get it up, smoking has drastically reduced your sperm count.

5 Increase harmful cholesterol levels

Smoking puts you at high risk of blocked arteries and blood clots.

6 Suffocate you

Smoking replaces the oxygen in your bloodstream with carbon monoxide.

7 Destroy your lungs

Smoking causes irreparable damage to your lung tissue, giving you emphysema.

8 Destroy the thin layer of fat just underneath your skin

That haggard, greying look is so common in the heavy-smoking world of supermodels that makeup artists now call it 'smokers' skin'.

9 Cause gum disease

This leads to loose teeth, bleeding gums and halitosis.

10 Greatly increase your likelihood of heart disease and strokes

Do you STILL feel like smoking?

doctors are now allowed to write 'smoking' on a death certificate where it asks for cause. But if we know it's so bad for us, why do so many men smoke so enthusiastically? The answer to that is because it's so hard to give up.

In terms of addictive qualities, there is very little that crack cocaine could teach nicotine. If tobacco was new on the market today, there really is little doubt that nicotine would be regarded as a Class A drug, and that is not counting the enormous range of chemicals that are added to cigarettes to further enhance your cravings. As soon as you spark up, nicotine invades your bloodstream and rapidly affects your nervous system, increasing your heart rate and inducing an instant feeling of euphoria. But the feeling goes almost as quickly as it

arrives and from the moment you put out a cigarette you start to come down from that nicotine high and want another rush – which you can only get from another cigarette.

When you think you're feeling rubbish because you haven't had a smoke, you're actually feeling normal and are wanting to get high again. The problem is that nicotine tolerance increases fairly rapidly, so you have to smoke more to maintain the same rush, and the more you smoke the more the nicotine high comes to represent a normal state of affairs. One of the major psychological hurdles of giving up is coming to terms with the idea that how you feel without nicotine is how you're supposed to feel.

But it can be done.

Smokingski is good for you, niet?

World Health Authority figures for men over 15 who smoke by nation (early 1990s):

- Russia 67%
- Turkey 63%
- Japan 59%
- Cuba 49.3%
- Israel 45%
- France 40%
- Germany 36.8%
- Canada 31%
- USA 28.1%
- United Kingdom 28%
- Sweden 22%

How to give up

Nobody is going to pretend that giving up a drug as powerful and addictive as nicotine is going to be easy. As well as the physical cravings, cigarettes exert a strong psychological hold on a smoker because the action of smoking becomes so much a part of his life. However, thousands of people manage to quit every year, so it can be done. These simple commandments will help you get through it as painlessly as possible.

- Make up your mind, then fix a date to stop and make sure you do.

- When you do give up, stop dead. Although cutting down significantly – like not smoking during the day – can help, don't attempt to phase out cigarettes by going down to one or two a day. If you are going to do that, then simply quit.

- Don't do it at a particularly stressful time, like during exams or just before getting married or on the birth of a baby. Try to pick a time when you will be as relaxed as possible.

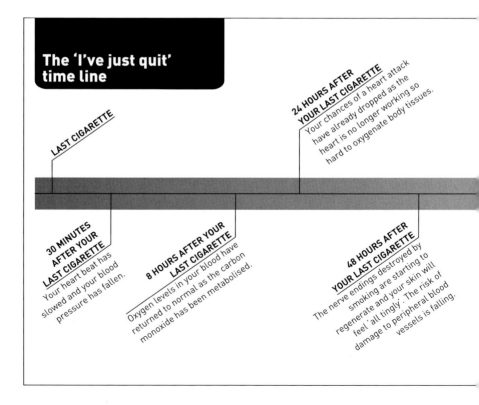

The 'I've just quit' time line

LAST CIGARETTE

24 HOURS AFTER YOUR LAST CIGARETTE
Your chances of a heart attack have already dropped as the heart is no longer working so hard to oxygenate body tissues.

30 MINUTES AFTER YOUR LAST CIGARETTE
Your heart beat has slowed and your blood pressure has fallen.

8 HOURS AFTER YOUR LAST CIGARETTE
Oxygen levels in your blood have returned to normal as the carbon monoxide has been metabolised.

48 HOURS AFTER YOUR LAST CIGARETTE
The nerve endings destroyed by smoking are starting to regenerate and your skin will feel 'all tingly'. The risk of damage to peripheral blood vessels is falling.

- Do it without aids such as patches or gum. Giving up smoking is all about willpower and too often people expect the patches or whatever to do the work for them, so they don't put in the mental effort. The re-offending rate among those who didn't use an aid is much lower than among those who did.

- Try not to tell people you are giving up. Although most of your friends will want to be supportive, it will become an irritatingly dominant topic of conversation: your progress, giving-up anecdotes, other people's fail-safe methods and so on. In the very early stages, when your cravings

are high and you are more than a little frazzled, these are the last things you want to talk about.

- Vary your routine. You'll have got into the habit of smoking in certain situations or at certain times of the day, so avoid getting into those circumstances and you will avoid a definite craving.

- Stay out of the bar, for a few weeks at least. The association of beer and fags will put a ridiculous strain on your resolve, and the more you have to drink the more you will weaken.

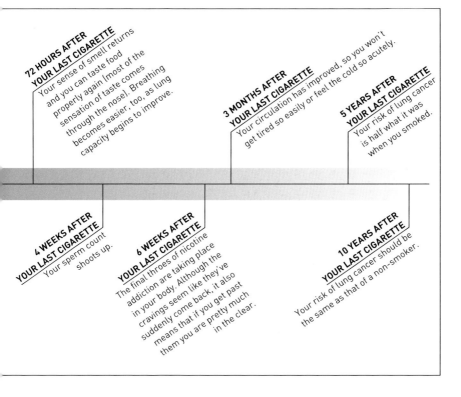

72 HOURS AFTER YOUR LAST CIGARETTE
Your sense of smell returns and you can taste food properly again (most of the sensation of taste comes through the nose). Breathing becomes easier, too, as lung capacity begins to improve.

3 MONTHS AFTER YOUR LAST CIGARETTE
Your circulation has improved, so you won't get tired so easily or feel the cold so acutely.

5 YEARS AFTER YOUR LAST CIGARETTE
Your risk of lung cancer is half what it was when you smoked.

4 WEEKS AFTER YOUR LAST CIGARETTE
Your sperm count shoots up.

6 WEEKS AFTER YOUR LAST CIGARETTE
The final throes of nicotine addiction are taking place in your body. Although the cravings seem like they've suddenly come back, it also means that if you get past them you are pretty much in the clear.

10 YEARS AFTER YOUR LAST CIGARETTE
Your risk of lung cancer should be the same as that of a non-smoker.

- Try not to hang out with smokers. Breathing secondary smoke will eventually trigger your nicotine addiction and your cravings will go through the roof – this is another good reason not to go to the bar until you're under control.

- Be prepared. Get rid of the smoking paraphernalia that reminds you of what you are missing. And as you will find yourself eating and snacking more, stock up on healthy, non-fattening stuff like fruit and raw veg. Try to avoid crisps and cakes.

- Don't worry about the weight gain. Your weight would have been artificially lowered before, as cigarettes speed up your metabolism. Besides, if you've got what it takes to give up smoking, losing a bit of fat later on will be nothing or, at least, much easier than living with a selection of smoke-related ailments.

- Drink plenty of water. It helps to flush toxins out of your system.

- Take each day at a time. When you give up, set your sights on going that morning without a snout, then try to get to the evening and after that concentrate on making it through to bedtime. Then aim at making the whole of the next day smoke free. And the next. After that, see if you can make it to the end of the week.

Cigars aren't safe

Giving up cigarettes in favour of a pipe or cigars might seem like a safe option because you don't inhale – well, it isn't. Safer, yes, but safe, no. Your lungs may be less exposed to smoke, but you are still running a major risk of cancer of the mouth, throat and larynx, and of contracting chronic conditions like bronchitis and emphysema. Also, bear in mind the amount of smoking you are doing with a decent-sized pipe or a respectable cigar – it may take over an hour to finish, the same time it would take to smoke about a dozen cigarettes. And do spare a thought for those around you and consider the sheer volume of secondary smoke given off by a cigar or pipe, which will be breathed in just as riskily.

- Reward yourself. But not with a big cigar! Save the money you would have spent on cigs and, after a set amount of time, use it to treat yourself to something you've always wanted.

Outside help

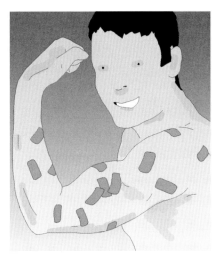

Although, ultimately, you need to give up smoking for yourself, there are accepted avenues you can go down for assistance.

HYPNOTHERAPY

Hypnosis puts you into a deeply relaxed, trance-like state, during which the therapist introduces the suggestion that you do not want to smoke again. Some people find afterwards that smoke in the mouth triggers the sensation of a very bad taste. Hypnotherapy is a reasonably successful method of giving up smoking and research has shown around a 35 per cent hit rate of people that kick the habit. It is, however, shrouded in smoke (dry ice) and mirrors, so be very careful before parting with your cash as there are many charlatans operating in the Give Up Smoking Instantly arena. Either go by personal recommendation or go to your doctor for advice.

Nicotine patches are not a good fashion statement. It is better to try giving up without them.

NICOTINE SUBSTITUTES

Nicotine patches, chewing gum and inhalers are cleverly designed to administer a steadily decreasing dose of nicotine until it is totally phased out by the end of a prescribed period (usually one month). It is best to get advice from your doctor or pharmacist before starting out on a course of nicotine substitutes, but if the instructions are followed carefully this method can be reasonably successful in dealing with your physical nicotine addiction. Why people using substitutes have such woeful re-offending rates is because these products do not address the psychological aspects of your smoking habit, so it will still be tough to give up. Remember, if you revert to smoking, stop using the substitutes immediately or there is a real danger you could OD on nicotine, which could have a serious effect on your heart.

ACUPUNCTURE

This ancient branch of Chinese healing involves inserting needles under the skin at various prescribed points to clear the blocked channels through which a person's life force (chi) flows. Usually acupuncture is used to treat chronic pain, but the therapy's success rate in curing addictions – smoking included – is pretty good. However, it does take a leap of faith to submit to something that makes no logical sense and involves needles. Make sure you go to an accredited acupuncturist (see local press for contacts), but be warned – such is the soothing power of these Chinese needles that people often get addicted to acupuncture itself.

Every breath you take

There is no point in taking care of your heart if you neglect your lungs. Lurking within your ribcage, these are the bellows that supply the oxygen that gets pumped around your body, and they are every bit as sensitive as your pump is.

Your lungs are much abused – given the degree of 21st-century air pollution and the rising figures for smoking – but they are absolutely vital for a healthy and active life. For any sort of life, actually. Put very simply, your lungs expand to take in oxygen from the atmosphere and contract to expel carbon dioxide, the waste produced when oxygen is used by the body's tissues. And, really, there isn't much more to it than that, but knowing how the respiratory system operates will help enormously when it comes to understanding how to keep your lungs healthy and functioning to their fullest efficiency.

The lungs are powered by the diaphragm, a large, strong muscle that is the floor of your chest cavity, and by the muscles between the ribs (the intercostal muscles). Breathing is under the control of the brain, which sends constant impulses to these muscles, making them alternately contract and relax to alter the size of the chest cavity. For inward breaths, the diaphragm and intercostal muscles contract, expanding the chest cavity and lungs and allowing air to be drawn in. When the muscles relax, the lungs contract, pushing air out. The brain automatically regulates the rate and extent of the diaphragm's movement by working out how much oxygen your system needs at a particular time. This means your breathing alters, becoming faster/slower or deeper/shallower to meet requirements.

When the lungs expand, oxygen is drawn into the system through the mouth or nose and flows into the part of the upper respiratory tract known as the trachea, or windpipe. From here, the tract divides into the two major airways, the right and left bronchi, which supply each of the lungs. Within the lungs, each bronchus branches out into thousands of progressively smaller pathways known as bronchioles, which end

Breath-taking facts about taking breath

Healthy adult men take between 12 and 15 breaths per minute.

During sleep, this rate drops to around 10 breaths per minute, but they will be deeper.

Strenuous exercise or stress should raise the breathing rate to 20 or more breaths per minute.

Under normal conditions, the complete cycle of each breath lasts about five seconds, but this will be shorter during exercise and longer during sleep.

Each breath takes in approximately 0.5 cubic litres (30 cu in) of air, and this can increase to up to four times as much during exertion.

The lungs

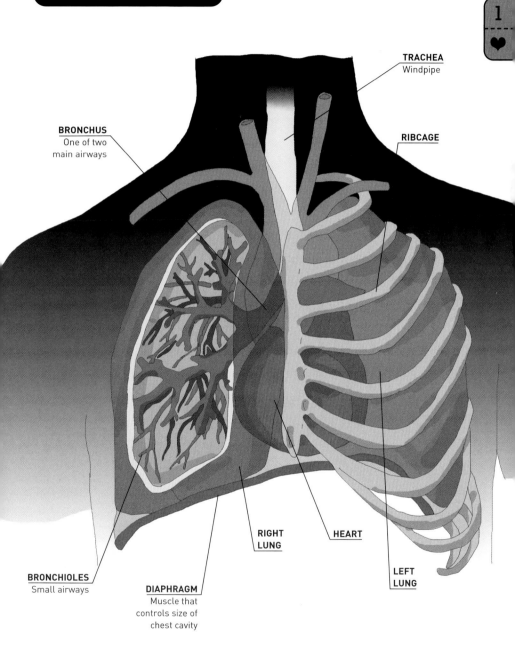

TRACHEA
Windpipe

BRONCHUS
One of two
main airways

RIBCAGE

**RIGHT
LUNG**

HEART

**LEFT
LUNG**

BRONCHIOLES
Small airways

DIAPHRAGM
Muscle that
controls size of
chest cavity

in clusters of tiny air sacs called alveoli. The lungs are not two large air pockets, like balloons, but have an internal structure more like a honeycomb or a sponge, made up of an enormous number of these tiny airbags, which inflate and contract in concert.

The exchange of oxygen and carbon dioxide takes place in the alveoli. Oxygen passes through the walls of the alveoli (which are very, very thin) and is taken into the network of capillaries (tiny blood vessels) surrounding the alveoli. As oxygen enters the bloodstream, carbon dioxide passes from the blood in the opposite direction, being taken into the alveoli and then exhaled from the lungs through the nose or mouth.

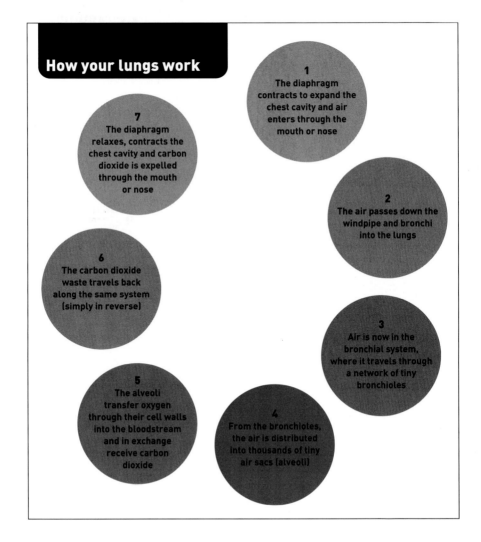

How your lungs work

1
The diaphragm contracts to expand the chest cavity and air enters through the mouth or nose

7
The diaphragm relaxes, contracts the chest cavity and carbon dioxide is expelled through the mouth or nose

2
The air passes down the windpipe and bronchi into the lungs

6
The carbon dioxide waste travels back along the same system (simply in reverse)

3
Air is now in the bronchial system, where it travels through a network of tiny bronchioles

5
The alveoli transfer oxygen through their cell walls into the bloodstream and in exchange receive carbon dioxide

4
From the bronchioles, the air is distributed into thousands of tiny air sacs (alveoli)

Breathe easily

There are a number of common respiratory system ailments, most of which are easily avoided or dealt with.

UPPER RESPIRATORY TRACT INFECTIONS

These affect the sinuses, larynx (voice box), nose and throat, and include colds, laryngitis, tonsillitis, sinusitis and pharyngitis. Most of these infections are not serious, causing no more than a sore throat or that bunged-up feeling, and can be taken care of with rest or in some cases a course of antibiotics. It is worth remembering that, in spite of what your mum used to say, you don't catch a cold by getting cold – it's a virus and feeling shivery is simply one of the symptoms.

LOWER RESPIRATORY TRACT INFECTIONS

These are more serious, and occur in the trachea, the bronchi and the lungs. Perhaps the most worrying is pneumonia, which is an inflammation of the lungs caused by an infection. Most types of pneumonia are the result of either a viral or a bacterial infection, but a significant number of cases are the result of a foreign body bringing infection into the lungs – inhaled vomit, drink or food are common causes, and it is not unusual to get pneumonia as a side effect of prolonged cocaine snorting. Pneumonia is usually treatable with medication, although in extreme cases the lungs may need mechanical help to function and expel excess mucus.

The other main lower respiratory tract infection is bronchitis, an inflammation of the lining of the bronchi, which can occur as the

You will be particularly susceptible to breathing problems if ...

- You smoke.
- You spend a lot of time in a smoke-filled environment.
- You live in an area heavily polluted with smog or traffic fumes.
- Your work involves a great deal of dust or tiny airborne particles.
- Your work involves chemicals in the area – dry cleaners are at particular risk.
- Your home is not sufficiently ventilated.
- You snort cocaine or any other powder.

See your doctor if ...

The following are the most obvious symptoms of lung disorder, and if any of them persist you should consult a healthcare professional:

Coughing
If it is persistent or persistently deep.

Mucus
If you are coughing up mucus that is yellow, deep green or brown.

Breathlessness
If you can't catch your breath under normal circumstances (not during or after physical exertion).

Wheezing
Normal breathing is more or less silent; be concerned if you hear or feel internal wheezing or whistling.

Chest pains
If breathing in or out, or coughing hurts.

---

result of a viral or bacterial infection. Bronchitis causes congestion of the airways through excess mucus production, leading to coughing and tightness of the chest. Prolonged exposure to outside pollutants can also cause bronchitis, and smoking is a major factor in the chronic, or long-term, form of the ailment. Bronchitis usually clears up by itself. If it is caused by external irritants, these must be avoided, while inhaling steam or menthol vapours can relieve the symptoms by warming and humidifying the airways and so loosening bronchial obstructions.

LUNG CANCER

Top of the table for causing cancer deaths among men, lung cancer is the most common form of cancer in in the UK. The disease is responsible for over 30,000 deaths a year, nearly all of people over the age of 40, with between 65 and 75 the peak ages.

The most common cause of lung cancer is smoking – the more you smoke and the younger you started being directly relative to your chances of getting the disease. Secondary smoking, high levels of pollution and working with asbestos or radiation account for about 20 per cent of lung cancer cases.

Prolonged exposure to the chemicals in tobacco smoke affects cells in the lungs and they begin to multiply uncontrollably, forming malignant tumours that can spread to destroy large areas of lung tissue. The cancer can also spread beyond the lungs, via the bloodstream, to other parts of the body such as the liver and the brain. The damaged tissues will show up on a chest X-ray as a dark shadow on the lungs, and a biopsy (the removal of a minute piece of tissue for examination) will confirm exactly what it is.

Treatments for lung cancer include radiotherapy, chemotherapy and sometimes surgery, in which part of or a whole lung is removed. Although surgery, if it is early enough, increases the lung cancer survival rate, overall only eight per cent of patients survive more than five years beyond their diagnosis.

EMPHYSEMA

Another side effect of smoking, this is when the walls of the tiny alveoli in the lungs become hardened by chemicals in cigarette smoke. Over time, the damage causes extreme shortage of breath. Emphysema inhibits the passage of oxygen into the bloodstream, which eventually results in a serious shortage of oxygen in the blood and puts considerable strain on the heart as it tries to compensate. Emphysema cannot be cured and the damage to the alveoli is irreversible.

PLEURISY

The pleura is a double-layered membrane that lies between the outside of the lungs and the inside of the chest cavity. Pleurisy is an inflammation of the membrane, most often caused by an infection that has spread from the lungs (pneumonia, for instance). This can cause considerable discomfort, including sharp chest pains when you breathe in. Pleurisy may be relieved with anti-inflammatory drugs but the underlying complaint also needs to be treated.

TUBERCULOSIS

Also known as TB or consumption, this bacterial infection is more associated with Victorian slums than the 21st century but, thanks to a new strain of bacteria, it is becoming worryingly prevalent today. In spite of that, TB doesn't seem to have nearly the

Clean-up act

Although the air around us will almost inevitably be full of the sort of foreign bodies we don't want ending up in our lungs, the respiratory system operates its own series of filters. Your nose contains thousands of tiny hairs that remove the larger airborne particles, which is why, when you were a kid, you were always being told to breathe through it! Further along, the trachea and bronchial tubes are lined with minuscule fibres called cilia, which catch smaller pollutants such as those found in cigarette smoke. Cells in the bronchi also produce a sticky mucus that traps irritants and is expelled by the reflex action of coughing once it has built up. These cells react to pollution in the pipes and produce increasing amounts of mucus as needed, which is why you automatically start coughing when you enter a polluted atmosphere.

same mortality rate as 100 years ago and the vast majority of people who are infected are unaware of it. Only the more extreme cases result in coughing, chest pains, breathlessness or fatigue, and fatalities are rare. TB is spread by airborne infection – coughing, sneezing, laughing or even sighing are enough for an infected person to pass it on. The bacteria are taken into the lungs where, if the immune system doesn't destroy them, they cause tissue damage and a build-up of fluid. In most cases the disease is not detected unless the person is specifically tested for it, and frequently people find out they have TB only when they are being treated for something else. The infection can be cured with long-term drug treatment. The best defence is the BCG vaccination.

Asthma

One in 20 of the population of the UK suffers from asthma and the rates are rising throughout the Western world. The condition is more common in children than among adults. The symptoms of an asthma attack include wheezing, coughing and a tightness in the chest that leads to a sudden shortness of breath. During an attack, the walls of the bronchi (the tubes that deliver air to the lungs) constrict, shutting off the air supply to the lungs. To make matters worse, the linings of the tubes swell up, triggering increased mucus production – the system's natural reaction to a blockage – further adding to the obstruction. As the body is starved of oxygen, the sufferer may experience a rapid heartbeat, sweating and feelings of panic.

The usual cause of asthma that starts in childhood is an over-sensitive reaction of the respiratory system to certain inhaled substances (allergens), and the condition is often inherited. When asthma starts in adulthood, there is often no obvious cause. There is no cure for asthma as such. The condition has to be 'managed' by avoiding the circumstances that bring on attacks (see list on the right) and working closely with your healthcare professional to take advantage of every available preventive measure. Inhalers are a commonly used method of instantly alleviating an attack by delivering a blast of an airway-opening bronchodilator drug. Oral drugs are sometimes recommended for long-term preventive treatment.

COMMON CAUSES OF ASTHMA

Allergens

Pollen, house dust, animal fur or feathers are the most common triggers. (In sufficient amounts, these irritants would affect even the healthiest respiratory system, but in asthma sufferers the body over-reacts.)

Exercise

Anything that puts a strain on the cardiovascular system either very suddenly or for an extended period of time.

Air pollution

Smoke, smog, fumes, car exhausts, chemical sprays and so on.

Weather conditions

Sudden blasts of cold air or swift barometric pressure changes can cause the airways to react.

Stress

Anxiety attacks or sudden stress can disrupt the breathing.

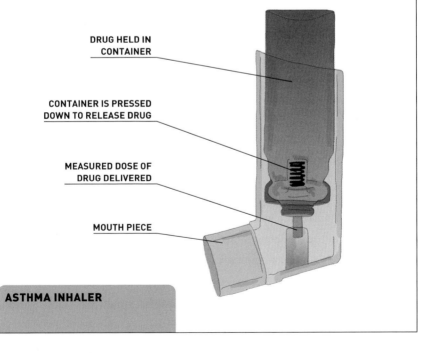

DRUG HELD IN CONTAINER

CONTAINER IS PRESSED DOWN TO RELEASE DRUG

MEASURED DOSE OF DRUG DELIVERED

MOUTH PIECE

ASTHMA INHALER

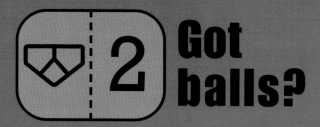

2 Got balls?

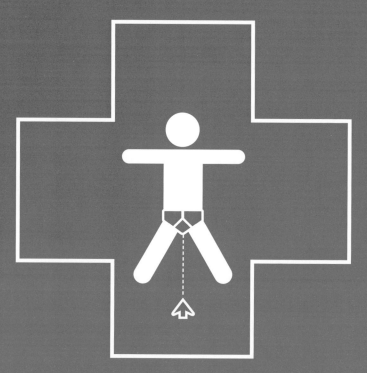

BECAUSE OF HOW THE MEDIA AND THE ENTERTAINMENT INDUSTRY PRESENT THINGS THESE DAYS, WE GET THE MESSAGE THAT MANY OF MODERN MAN'S PROBLEMS ARE SEXUALLY ORIENTED. BUT AS FAR AS THE PRACTICALITIES GO, HAVING A HAPPY AND HEALTHY SEX LIFE IS PRETTY STRAIGHTFORWARD.

Where do babies come from?

Every man knows what his penis and his scrotum looks like and feels like, but surprisingly few know what goes on inside.

Man's reproductive system is not only a source of pleasure, it is also a masterpiece of engineering: the testes are hung outside the body to keep them cooler; the penis is erect only when it's being called into action; and the same tube is used to deliver both urine and semen, yet they don't get mixed up.

The testes, the walnut-sized solids that can be felt inside the scrotal sac, are where sperm are produced in coils of minute tubes – which would stretch 500 metres (1650 feet) if unravelled – and stored until needed.

The man's participation in the reproductive cycle begins on sexual arousal, when the penis becomes erect (see pages 74–75) and a small amount of fluid is secreted over its tip to clean away any traces of urine from the urethra in preparation for ejaculation. While this is going on, the testes swell to nearly twice their normal size, and from each one sperm is pushed up through a tube called the vas deferens and into a reservoir, the ejaculatory duct, ready to go into action.

Meanwhile, the prostate gland and two small sacs called the seminal vesicles produce semen, the milky grey fluid that the sperm swim in on their journey to the woman's fallopian tubes, where an egg might be waiting. Semen and sperm mingle as they enter the urethra and on orgasm travel up the penis for ejaculation.

During orgasm, a series of sharp contractions tighten muscles in the buttocks

Over the past two decades sperm count in the Western world has fallen dramatically. Experts believe that an officially infertile level is going to be reached very soon. Forget meteors from outer space, forget hostile aliens or freak tidal waves: the end of the world is in your pants, so be warned.

and stomach, and around the base of the penis, forcing sperm out under pressure.

The deep waves of pleasure men experience at orgasm occur not only because the nerves that supply the genital area spread a tingling sensation over many parts of the body, but also because pleasure-producing chemicals are released in the brain. Very soon after ejaculation, the muscles around and in the penis relax and the erection fades.

And then you fall asleep, a very happy man. But you really should cuddle her for a bit, just to show willing.

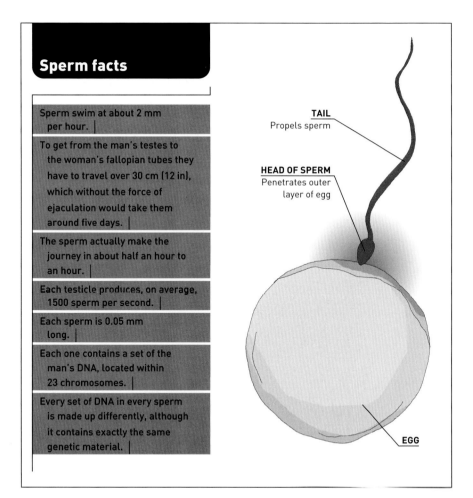

Sperm facts

Sperm swim at about 2 mm per hour.

To get from the man's testes to the woman's fallopian tubes they have to travel over 30 cm (12 in), which without the force of ejaculation would take them around five days.

The sperm actually make the journey in about half an hour to an hour.

Each testicle produces, on average, 1500 sperm per second.

Each sperm is 0.05 mm long.

Each one contains a set of the man's DNA, located within 23 chromosomes.

Every set of DNA in every sperm is made up differently, although it contains exactly the same genetic material.

TAIL
Propels sperm

HEAD OF SPERM
Penetrates outer layer of egg

EGG

What's the deferens to you?

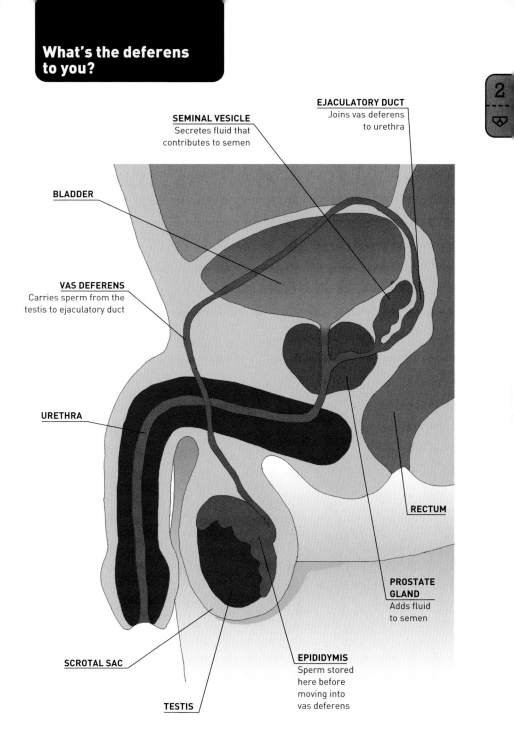

EJACULATORY DUCT
Joins vas deferens
to urethra

SEMINAL VESICLE
Secretes fluid that
contributes to semen

BLADDER

VAS DEFERENS
Carries sperm from the
testis to ejaculatory duct

URETHRA

RECTUM

**PROSTATE
GLAND**
Adds fluid
to semen

SCROTAL SAC

EPIDIDYMIS
Sperm stored
here before
moving into
vas deferens

TESTIS

2

In the immortal words of the great Woody Allen: 'Sex and death are two things that should happen to a man at least once in his life.'
Make sure that one is not followed by the other and practice safe sex at all times.
Know your lover well and know their medical history.
When in doubt, wear a condom.

Coming too soon?

Premature ejaculation is pretty normal: it's the most common sexual complaint in the UK, as one-third of all men experience it at some time in their lives. There is no 'cure' in the accepted sense, because there isn't really any easily identifiable cause. There is rarely any physical reason behind it, and even the circumstances in which it happens appear to be completely random – thus it is very difficult to address. Indeed, premature ejaculation seems almost entirely psychological, due to unrelated stress, difficulties elsewhere within a relationship, nervousness, anticipation, fear of discovery, worries about performance or even over-excitement about having sex with a particular partner. The best ways to cope with the problem are not to be ashamed, to talk it over immediately with your partner – who should be sympathetic – and to relax. Ironically, one of the biggest factors in premature ejaculation is worrying about premature ejaculation. Make the whole act of love-making less focused on pen-etration, and bring your partner to orgasm in other ways.

The strange case of the disappearing sperm

Over the last couple of decades, the sperm count of men in the Western world has been falling steadily: the number of sperm per millilitre (ml) has dropped from 100 million/ml to around half that, at between 50 and 60 million/ml. Given that a sperm count of under 40 million/ml is considered to be below the ideal level for efficient fertility and below 20 million/ml is considered infertile, this isn't a healthy trend. It's made worse by the fact that what sperm are produced are much less mobile than they were 30 years ago; and the volume of semen produced by modern man has almost halved in that time.

Worryingly low sperm counts (below 30 million/ml) affect around 1.2 million men in the UK; infertility affects about 15 per cent of all men and nearly half of them will seek treatment. Environmental pollution is believed to be the main cause of this drop in sperm rates, as DDT and other pesticides that are now part of our food chain have the same effect on the human body as the female hormone oestrogen. Lifestyle changes in that we drink more, smoke more and work harder for longer hours are thought to contribute, too.

Although this reduction in sperm count and quality has yet to reach the point at which it will threaten the human race – between 10 million/ml and 20 million/ml is still 30 per cent

efficient – it shouldn't be ignored. It is worth finding out how to maximise your sperm count, especially if you and your partner are trying to conceive.

FOR A HIGHER SPERM COUNT

Give up smoking and reduce the toxins in your system.

Don't smoke weed – there are direct links between sustained cannabis use and low sperm counts.

If you are overweight lose some fat; it will redress your hormone balance.

Cut down on drinking – more than five units a day will drastically and immediately reduce sperm count.

Don't drink so much coffee.

Keep your testicles cool – showers are better than hot baths.

Relax: long-term stress can adversely affect your sperm count.

Eat organic, pesticide-free produce.

Making a stand

Erections are part of a man's life from puberty onwards, but at no time will he be in control of them.

When something happens that turns you on – you see something, touch something, read something or think about something that you find very sexy – then the chances are you'll feel a tingle in your loins, the beginnings of an erection. Your brain has started to trigger a set of responses that are all about man's primal urge to reproduce. We are programmed to have sex, it's one of our most basic instincts.

The sequence begins when the brain takes on board an image or sensation it perceives to be erotic; exactly what this might be is a highly individual matter of learned personal taste and preference. The brain sends a series of impulses to the nerves around the base of the penis – this is what causes the tingling in the loins – and they relax the muscles within the walls of the arteries that run the length of the shaft. This slackening allows the spongy tissues inside the penis to fill up with blood, and the pressure makes the penis rigid.

The penis has three internal chambers. Two, known as the corpora cavernosa, are where the main force behind the erection takes place. These run the entire length of the penis and consist of tissues, blood vessels and empty spaces that accommodate the extra blood. A smaller chamber, the corpus spongiosum, is situated on the underside of the penis and surrounds the urethra to prevent damage or interference; this, too, fills with blood.

The more blood flowing into the penis, the harder the erection. The blood is prevented from flowing out of the tissues again by pressure on the veins leading from the engorged tissues. As long as the penis remains stimulated it automatically maintains the erection. Once orgasm is achieved or stimulus ceases, the brain stops sending messages to the nerves around the base of the penis, the muscles in the artery walls contract and the erection starts to deflate. As it does so, the pressure is taken off the veins, removing any obstruction to the outflow of blood.

What goes up must first get up

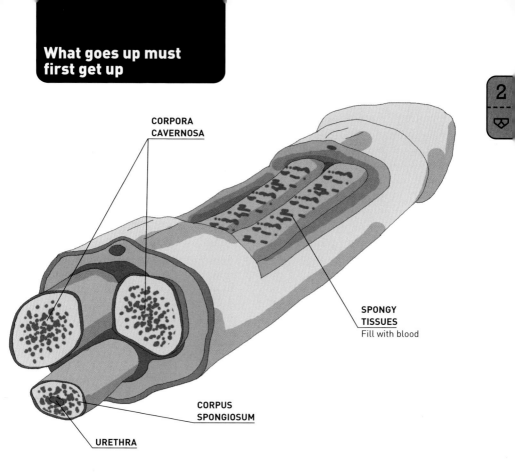

CORPORA CAVERNOSA

SPONGY TISSUES
Fill with blood

CORPUS SPONGIOSUM

URETHRA

Morning glory

Flattering as it might be for your partner, that early morning erection has got little to do with arousal and more to do with needing the loo. On average, men get three or four erections during the course of a night, each lasting around half an hour, and the last one may be maintained if a full bladder prevents blood from flowing out of the penis. As the night goes on the bladder gradually fills up and when it gets to a certain size it presses on the tissues at the base of the penis, preventing the erection-forming blood from draining away. As soon you start to empty your bladder the erection begins to deflate.

Don't be soft

Erectile dysfunction affects every man at some point in his life, and the trick is not to let it, er, get you down.

It would be wrong to say it is all in the mind, but the main causes of erectile dysfunction are psychological. The situation is not unlike premature ejaculation in one respect – stressing about not being able to get an erection is the most likely thing to prevent it happening. Worry about what is going on outside the bedroom won't help either, as stress and anxiety about other aspects of your life are liable to manifest themselves in a potentially embarrassing droop. Depressive illness can contribute, too, as can the cold stark fact that you might not fancy the person you are with as much as you thought you did. On this note, rows and problems within long-term relationships can sometimes lead to bedtime flaccidity, which, if the idea was make-up sex, isn't going to help matters.

There are, of course, two famous, self-inflicted physical causes of regular erectile dysfunction: smoking and drinking. Brewer's droop isn't a myth – sustained heavy drinking not only affects your sperm count but also your ability to have an erection. Cigarette smoking interferes with the circulation to such a degree that it can affect the blood flow into the penis. Other physical causes of erectile dysfunction are less easily avoidable. Diabetes is a big one, as a quarter of young diabetic men have problems getting an erection, a figure that rises to nearer three-quarters for diabetics over the age of 60. Spinal cord injuries can result in impotence, while the circulatory diseases that clog up the arteries and limit blood flow are a major cause of erectile dysfunction among older men.

To find out if your difficulties are psychological or not, attempt to get an erection by masturbating – if you can, then it's nothing physical. The best things to do are not to worry, keep yourself fit, don't drink too much and give up smoking.

Saddle baggage

Research in the USA and in Norway has shown that while cycling may be very good for the cardiovascular system and improved health in general, it can have a negative effect on your erection. Competitive cyclists were found to have a much higher rate of erectile dysfunction than other similarly active sportsmen, figures that were directly related to how long they spent in the saddle. It seems the cyclists' weight constricted blood flow into their penises to such a degree that it frequently caused numbness and the inability to raise a satisfactory erection. The size of the saddle was a contribution too: slimline racing saddles were nearly three times as likely to cause erectile dysfunction as soft, fat saddles.

The happy pill

It's a miracle cure for impotence ... It's in the punchline of so many jokes ...
It's acquired a nightclub value as a recreational drug ...
But, really, what is Viagra?

It's sildenafil, an oral medication that came on the market in the USA in 1998. The drug was designed to help men with erectile problems by blocking the enzyme that interferes with the body's production of a hormone called cyclic guanosine monophosphate (cGMP), which helps to regulate blood flow into and out of the penis.

As you need to be sexually aroused before your body produces cGMP, and Viagra does nothing to increase production, the drug works only if you are sexually aroused to start off with. So don't worry about a permanent erection.

Viagra is not an aphrodisiac and will not get you aroused with partners you just don't fancy – it won't save a dead relationship.

The drug takes about half an hour to have an effect and 50 mg tablets (the most common dosage) usually remain effective for four hours.

Side effects can include flushing, headaches, reduced blood pressure, blurred vision and, strangely, a slight blue-green colour-blindness.

Do not use Viagra if you have been taking amyl nitrate for a heart condition, or any other prescription medication containing nitrates.

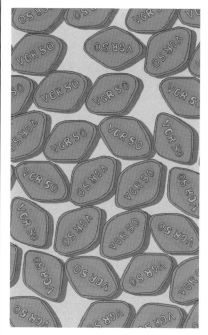

Actually, Viagra tablets are usually blue, but we couldn't afford to use any other colours.

Sexually transmitted diseases

In spite of recent high-profile sexual health campaigns, incidences of sexually transmitted diseases (STDs) continue to rise. Most of these infections remain avoidable.

At present, between one and two per cent of men a year in the UK get treatment for a sexually transmitted disease. That percentage is higher than it used to be and the rise shows no sign of slowing down. Nobody's exactly sure why, in the light of all that has been done to raise awareness of the issue during the last ten years, these rates are continuing to go up. A younger start to sexual activity and an increase in casual sex are cited as part of the reason but, perversely, another factor is that the public information campaign that did a great deal to raise HIV awareness was a little too successful. It is thought that many men – especially sexually naive youngsters – have come to believe that HIV is the only STD. Rightly or wrongly, they think that they are not in the high-risk group and therefore are less likely to need to take precautions. This is far from the case, however, and other sexually transmitted diseases are rising faster than HIV. All of the following can be caught and passed on by both men and women who practise unsafe sex.

CHLAMYDIA

This can cause infertility in women and be passed on to an unborn child, while in men, if untreated, can lead to a painful infection of the urethra. Symptoms in men include a burning sensation during urination, itching around the penis opening and a gunky discharge noticeable first thing in the morning. Women are less likely to show symptoms. It is treatable with antibiotics.

CRABS

Also known as pubic lice, these are small grey or brown insects that settle in the pubic hair and lay eggs at the base of each hair shaft. Sometimes, they can cause itching around the genital area. Crabs can be contracted from an infected sexual partner or from sleeping in an infected person's bed. They are dealt with by using a specially medicated shampoo (ordinary soap or shampoos will not work).

GENITAL HERPES

This is an infection by the herpes virus (one strain of which is also responsible for cold sores around the mouth). The symptoms are sore patches on the skin around the genitals, which lead to small circular blisters on a larger area of the buttocks, thighs and sexual

Despite the onset of AIDs in the 1980s, incidences of sexually transmitted diseases continue to rise at an alarming rate throughout the Western world.

GONORRHEA

A highly contagious bacterial infection, gonorrhea is far more common and easily spread than people realise. Around 7500 cases are diagnosed each year at STD clinics in the UK. A man has a 20 per cent chance of catching gonorrhea from the first sexual contact with an infected women, while a woman has a 90 per cent chance of catching it from an infected man. Symptoms are very painful urination accompanied by a discharge of pus, occasionally blood-flecked, from the penis or vagina. The infection can cause inflammation of the rectum or throat if contracted through anal or oral sex. If recognised early enough, gonorrhea can be cleared up with a single dose of antibiotics. If allowed to progress unchecked, it can cause inflammation of the urethra, prostate or the testicles and sometimes leads to infertility.

SYPHILIS

While the rate of syphilis infection in the UK has declined steeply in the last 20 years, and has vanished almost completely among heterosexuals, in the US it has recently been rising. This bacterial infection is a potentially very dangerous disease that invades the whole body, with symptoms of ulcers around the genitals, a widespread rash, hair loss and swollen glands. Syphilis is curable with penicillin, but if left untreated the infection can lie dormant in the body for years before flaring up without warning, destroying tissues and possibly causing mental illness.

HIV INFECTION AND AIDS

The human immunodeficiency virus (HIV) enters the body through contact with body fluids, including blood, saliva, semen or vaginal secretions. The virus weakens the

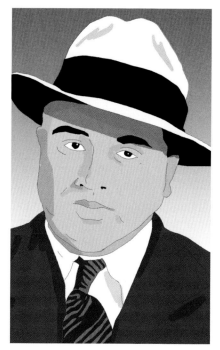

The American gangster Al Capone. The renowned and feared boss of the Mob, he sprayed his machine gun too often and died of syphilis.

organs. These can spread and open up to cause messy, painful sores. Antiviral drugs will control the outbreak, but the virus remains in the body and once infected you are likely to have further attacks, which must be treated again.

GENITAL WARTS

A very common, highly contagious viral STD, genital warts show up as small soft growths on the tip of the penis (or in and around the vagina in women) and can spread to form ugly, lumpy masses. The infection often clears up by itself, but you may need to use prescription creams.

body's ability to fight off disease by destroying certain cells, known as CD4 cells, which are a vital part of the immune system. Many people infected with HIV may be completely without symptoms for a long time. However, once the number of CD4 cells falls below a certain level – which can take up to ten years from the time of the infection – the immune system is pretty well useless and the sufferer is considered to have full-blown AIDS or acquired immunodeficiency syndrome. The initial signs of this include skin lesions, shingles, fatigue, weight loss, memory problems and a susceptibility to viral infections such as colds and flu. Later, serious diseases such as lung infections and cancers may develop. There is currently no cure for AIDS, although recently developed antiviral drugs may postpone the onset of the condition once HIV has been diagnosed.

AIDs has not only devastated Africa but is now making a significant scale of progress in China and Russia. Both countries are too poor and big to deal with the epidemic properly.

Sexual health

Technically, in the present day, the only form of completely safe sex is no sex at all. The advice given below is on safer sex practices that increase your chances of keeping healthy.

Use correctly fitting, kite-mark standard condoms; ill-fitting or weak rubbers are the most commonly cited cause of 'accidents'.

Don't use condoms that are past their expiry date and do not be tempted to reuse one, no matter if you have given it a good rinse out.

Be careful to put on a condom correctly.

Use only water-based lubricants with condoms, as oil-based jellies destroy latex.

Do not share sex toys.

Stay away from activities likely to cause bleeding, especially where there could be possible contact with semen.

Remember that STDs can be passed on by the fingers or the tongue or any other part of the body.

Don't forget, when you sleep with a new partner you are actually

sleeping with everybody else she
or he has slept with.

Be very careful when travelling
abroad; men are far more likely to
have unprotected sex with
strangers while on holiday than
they are at home.

Be wary when drunk. A large
number of unwanted pregnancies
involve both parties drinking
heavily before conception.

Try not to put it about more than
you have to. Regardless of
whether you believe you are
practising safe sex or not, your
chances of contracting an STD
go up as your number of
partners rises.

Get yourself checked out as soon
as you think you might have
contracted something; don't leave
it to get worse. Also, if you think
your partner might have passed
something on to you, then make
sure he or she has an
examination, too.

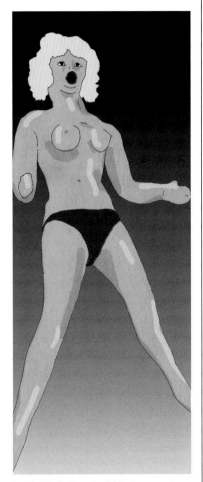

**Lovely Lilo is the only girl that you can be
really sure about after a night out.**

Prostate yourself

Sitting just beneath the bladder and right in front of the rectum, the prostate gland is a solid organ roughly the size and shape of a walnut. It surrounds the initial part of the uthera and produces a liquid that becomes part of seminal fluid during ejaculation. Only men have prostate glands.

Prostate Cancer

Although you will be unlikely to suffer from diagnosable prostate cancer until you are in your fifties, you're never too young to be aware of the tests that can be carried out to determine it.

DIGITAL RECTAL EXAMINATION

Since the prostate gland is so close to the rectum, the easiest way to feel for abnormality is for a doctor to insert a lubricated, gloved finger.

BLOOD OR URINE ANALYSIS

Specific tests have been developed to determine not only prostate cancer but any enlargement or inflammation of the gland.

ULTRASOUND SCANNING

It produces an image of the organ detailed enough to show any tumours.

The prostate gland starts to grow bigger during puberty, and will have reached its optimum size by the time you are in your early twenties. Prostate problems are extremely rare in men under the age of 30, and the two most common by far are prostate cancer and prostatitis (see page 83). Occasionally men over the age of 50 will experience further, apparently natural, growth of their prostate gland which has the effect of interfering with urination as it grows to compress the uthera and put pressure on the bladder. In extreme cases this will be treated with the removal of the prostate gland.

The cause of the third most common type of cancer among men (after lung cancer and bowel cancer), there are approximately 12,000 new cases of prostate cancer diagnosed every year in the UK. It is believed to be linked to high levels of testosterone, and occurs when a tumour, malignant or benign, forms on the outer layer of the prostate gland. There are relatively very few cases among men under 50 years old and although it can exist for several years before it reaches a diagnosable state, it rarely proves fatal.

Men over the age of 50 should have a prostate cancer examination once a year. However, if you are of African descent or have a history of prostate cancer in your family you are more susceptible, and should be annually screened from your mid-forties onwards.

The prostate gland

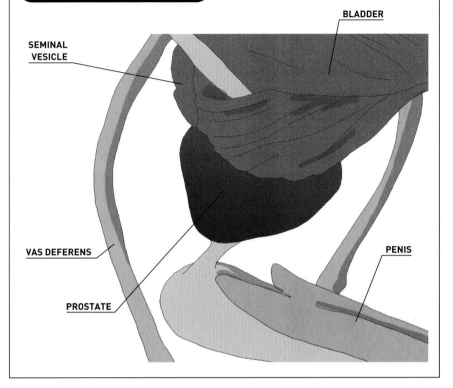

SEMINAL VESICLE

BLADDER

VAS DEFERENS

PENIS

PROSTATE

PROSTATITIS

Prostatitis is most likely to occur in men between the ages of 30 and 50, and unlike prostate cancer, it is a non-malignant inflammation of the prostate, and is divided into two types: bacterial and non-bacterial. The symptoms for each are the same and the effects are similar: a swelling of the prostate gland that becomes tender in itself and painful during urination. Even if it is only an inflamed prostate and not cancer, you will still have to brace yourself for a digital rectal examination and if the prostate is inflamed, samples of urine and secretion from the gland will be analysed to determine the type and cause.

The differences are in the treatment. As the former, and by far the most common form of prostatitis, is caused by the presence of bacteria it is treated with a course of antibiotics, which may last for as long as a month before the condition clears up. The latter will be treated with medication once whatever infection has caused the inflamation has been determined, while rest and painkillers should be taken to relieve the discomfort.

As a last resort, chronic prostatitis may be treated with surgery to remove the prostate gland.

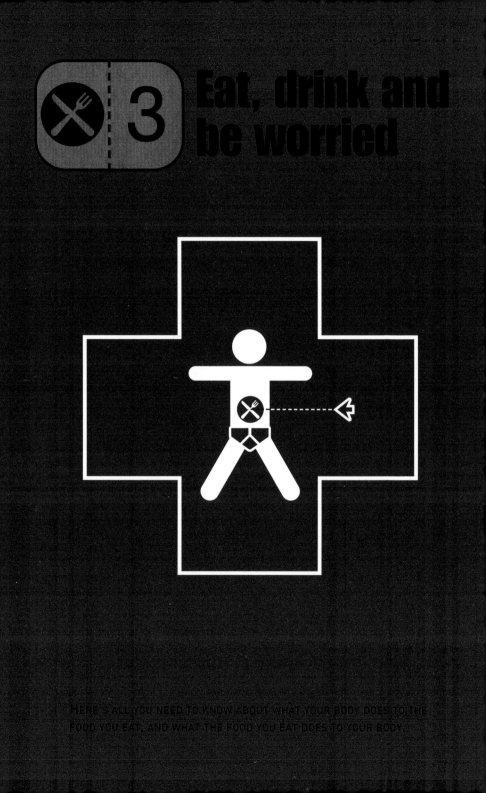

3 Eat, drink and be worried

HERE'S ALL YOU NEED TO KNOW ABOUT WHAT YOUR BODY DOES TO THE FOOD YOU EAT, AND WHAT THE FOOD YOU EAT DOES TO YOUR BODY.

Breakin' it down

The body extracts the nutrients we need from the food we eat by reducing it to its component parts. This takes place in a lot of tubes and chambers that are known as the digestive system.

Although it might seem that most of us live to eat, in fact it's the other way round and we eat to live. The whole primal purpose of us eating anything is to break food down to a sufficiently accessible state for the nutrients it contains to be absorbed by the system. Hunger comes upon us because we are running low on nutrients or carbo-hydrates to burn as fuel and those levels need topping up.

The food's journey through the digestive system begins in the mouth, where it is chewed up by the teeth and mixed with saliva to render it into a mass soft enough to be swallowed. This mass is pushed down into the oesophagus, where muscle contractions carry it on into the stomach. The average man's stomach has a capacity of 1–1½ litres (1½– 2½ pints) – it expands when full – and it acts as a holding pen, storing masticated food for several hours before releasing it into the small intestine. In the stomach, powerful acids begin to break the food down and destroy any bacteria, while muscles churn everything into a semi-liquid. Because of the time it takes for the small intestine to process food, the stomach has to hold on to its contents and release it in batches; otherwise you'd have to eat a small amount every quarter of an hour.

A grown man's small intestine is roughly 7 metres (23 feet) in length. As food is digested in this tube, it is propelled along from one section to the next by a series of muscular contractions. The initial section, about 0.5 metre (1½ feet) long, is the duodenum, where the molecules of the food

Nearly two-thirds of adults in the USA are overweight, and almost a third of them are obese, according to data from the 1999–2000 National Health and Nutrition Examination Survey. In 2001 it was calculated that some 40 million Americans were obese. Some 70 per cent of cases of cardiovascular disease in the country are a result of obesity.

Great guts!

If your digestive system is functioning efficiently then the rest of your body will be working much better too. Follow these simple guidelines and keep your guts healthy.

Drink at least 2 litres (3½ pints) of water a day.

Eat plenty of fibre, such as fruit and vegetables: between 25 and 30 grams a day is ideal.

Don't smoke.

Don't eat too much food prepared with flour – bread, pasta and so on.

Observe food hygiene guidelines.

Avoid cross-contamination in the kitchen – don't bring cooked and raw meat into contact with the same utensils.

Exercise daily.

to be digested – fats, carbs and protein – are broken down into smaller particles by digestive juices entering from the pancreas and gallbladder. Any iron, calcium or folic acid is absorbed into the system at this point. The next 3 metres (10 feet) of small intestine comprise the section called the jejunum, where the breakdown of nutrients is completed. By now, the food is a liquid containing a lot of water. In the remaining length of the small intestine, the ileum, the nutrients are absorbed into the body. This absorption occurs through the intestine walls as the nutrients pass into millions of tiny tendril-like projections called villi. The villi wave about from the inner intestinal wall and have a rich supply of blood that carries the nutrients into the system.

Any waste matter that hasn't been absorbed passes from the small intestine through to the large intestine, also known as the colon, by means of a one-way exit – the ileocaecal valve – which prevents any backflow. The large intestine, which is nearly 2 metres (6½ feet) long, absorbs water and some remaining vitamins and minerals into the system, leaving behind mainly indigestible fibre. This waste is compressed into faeces, or stools, which remain in the colon until expelled through the rectum.

The way the digestive system operates is incredibly complex – its functions are regulated by hormones and nerves, which work in collaboration to control the production of digestive juices and the rhythmic muscular contractions of the intestine walls. The digestive nervous system is actually more elaborate than that of the spinal column and carries out more functions than the brain during the course of a day.

The digestive system

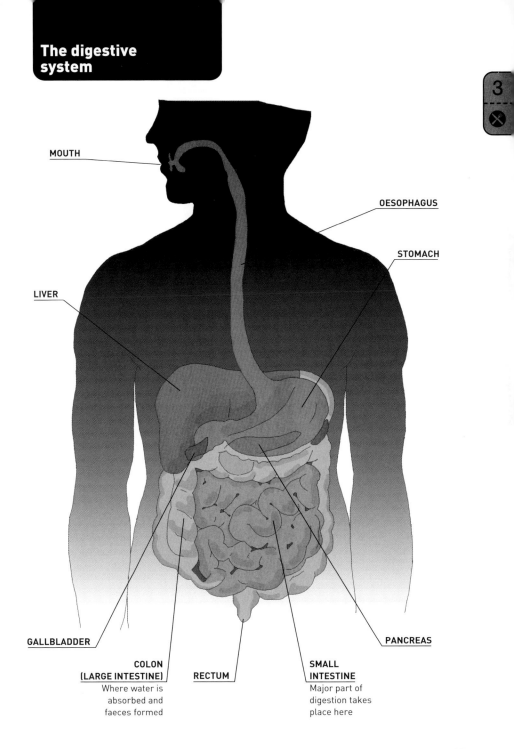

MOUTH

OESOPHAGUS

STOMACH

LIVER

GALLBLADDER

COLON
(LARGE INTESTINE)
Where water is
absorbed and
faeces formed

RECTUM

SMALL
INTESTINE
Major part of
digestion takes
place here

PANCREAS

3

The digestive clock

3

As you are probably aware, most foodstuffs that enter your body are in there for quite some time. This clock demonstrates how long it takes for a meal to be absorbed, used and expelled by your digestive system.

10 HOURS TO SEVERAL DAYS IN THE LARGE INTESTINE

The departure lounge. Waste products left behind after the main digestive process pass from the small intestine through to the large intestine, where they hang about waiting to be expelled through the rectum. How long they remain depends on the efficiency of your digestive system and the main components of the waste.

1–6 HOURS IN THE SMALL INTESTINE

Digestion is largely completed here, as this is where nutrients are absorbed into the bloodstream and fed to the various parts of the body. The length of time food spends in the small intestine depends on how quickly it can be broken down. Carbohydrates, for instance, break down quickly; some proteins can take for ever and you will be able to feel a decent-sized steak in your gut for many hours.

1–2 MINUTES IN THE MOUTH
It is chewed and broken down
to a consistency that makes it
easier to swallow.

**10 SECONDS IN
THE OESOPHAGUS**
It is swallowed into the
oesophagus, which is just a
passage into the stomach;
nothing actually happens here.

2–4 HOURS IN THE STOMACH
Food is reduced to a sludgy,
semi-liquid consistency in the
stomach by a combination of
natural digestive enzymes,
stomach acid and the churning
action of the stomach walls.

1

2

3

4

5

Ever wondered how long that burger you ate would be travelling around with you?

Bellyachin'

With a system as complex as the digestive tract, there is plenty that can go wrong. Most of it is short-lived or can be dealt with easily however, and a lot of problems are the result of dietary abuse, but some potential ailments are worth taking seriously.

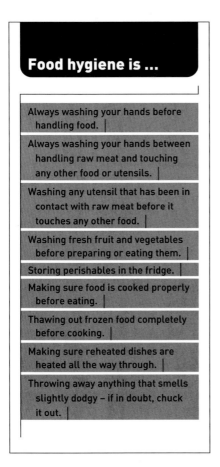

Food hygiene is ...

Always washing your hands before handling food.

Always washing your hands between handling raw meat and touching any other food or utensils.

Washing any utensil that has been in contact with raw meat before it touches any other food.

Washing fresh fruit and vegetables before preparing or eating them.

Storing perishables in the fridge.

Making sure food is cooked properly before eating.

Thawing out frozen food completely before cooking.

Making sure reheated dishes are heated all the way through.

Throwing away anything that smells slightly dodgy – if in doubt, chuck it out.

INDIGESTION

The medical term for this is dyspepsia, and it refers to any discomfort in the upper digestive system such as pain, nausea or wind. Men are more than twice as likely to suffer from it as women. Usually, the problem is caused by overloading the stomach, eating too quickly or while on the move, or eating rich or spicy foods, but it can also be caused by stress. Indigestion shouldn't last more than two or three hours and, in the short term, the symptoms can usually be relieved by taking antacid medicine or drinking milk. Constant indigestion can often be fixed by making lifestyle changes that allow you to eat your meals under more relaxed circumstances or by cutting out foods that clearly disagree with you. If, after making these changes, indigestion persists, you should see your doctor.

GASTRO-OESOPHAGEAL REFLUX DISEASE (GORD)

This refers to what happens when chewed food or stomach acid travels up the oesophagus from the stomach to the mouth, instead of in the other direction. It results in the hot pain known as heartburn and frequent belching. GORD can occur because the stomach is overfull or its muscles are malfunctioning and not closing the valve at the bottom properly, allowing acid or food to flow backwards. A condition called hiatus hernia, in which part of the stomach moves up into the chest, can be another cause of reflux. GORD is also often triggered by the ingestion of chocolate, peppermint, coffee,

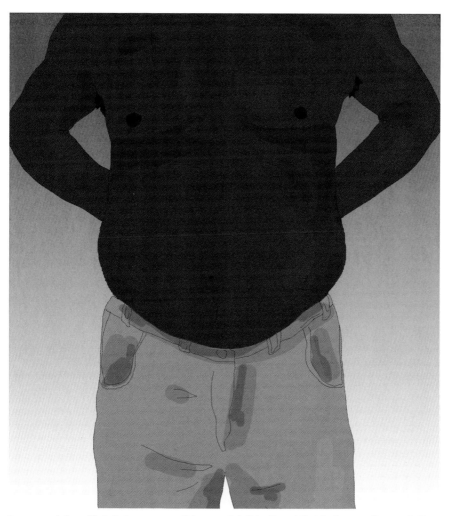

In some societies a big belly is seen as a religious symbol. Yet, although Buddha is generally accepted to have been a bit of a porker, you don't often see chubby Buddhist monks, do you?

alcohol, fruit juice or fat, and is more likely to occur in the obese than those of normal weight. If you suffer from frequent GORD attacks, the best ways to combat them are to cut back or give up the foods listed above, stop smoking, lose weight, eat frequent small meals rather than an occasional large one, and avoid bending over after eating.

PEPTIC ULCERS
A common digestive system complaint, peptic ulcers are on the rise thanks to our

speeded-up 21st-century lifestyle – more than one in ten people in the UK develop an ulcer during their lives. These ulcers occur when there is a breach in the layer of mucus that protects the lining of the stomach and upper intestine from the acids and digestive enzymes, and the corrosive acid comes into direct contact with the tissues. This can happen because of decreased mucus production, increased acid secretion, or outside irritants such as alcohol, caffeine or aspirin that attack the layer of mucus. Symptoms include burning abdominal pains, which may be relieved by eating, and bloating, nausea and gas. In spite of popular belief, ulcers are not caused by stress, but stressful situations can cause surges in stomach acid production that will irritate an existing ulcer. Peptic ulcers can be treated with drugs that lower the levels of stomach acid and allow the ulcer to heal itself, but to assist matters, sufferers should stop smoking, avoid drinking coffee, tea or alcohol, and eat more small meals during the day instead of one or two big ones.

Stay fit with fibre

Very few men in the UK and USA have anything like enough fibre in their diet. The recommended amount is between 18 and 24 grams per day, but the average British adult male consumes less than 12 grams. Fibre is one of the hardest working nutrients in the system: it keeps cholesterol levels in check; it can go a long way to stopping you overeating; and it can prevent your internal waste disposal system from shutting down.

There are two types of fibre you should be taking on board, soluble (as found in fruit, vegetables, cereals and pulses) and insoluble (whole grains and cereals, fruit and vegetable skins), which work in different ways. Soluble fibre slows down the digestion of glucose and other fats, meaning that after a rich meal cholesterol levels are less likely to rise suddenly and blood sugar spikes will be avoided (which is very important if you are diabetic) reducing post-feed fatigue. Soluble fibre also absorbs toxins found lurking in the digestive system. Insoluble fibre makes food chewier, which means you are likely to feel fuller quicker and so think you need to eat less. This type of fibre enormously reduces the chances of constipation as it is indigestible and adds solid volume to the waste matter that is passed into the colon, giving the intestinal muscles something to grip on and so expel waste far more efficiently.

Keep your friends close by taking an enema regularly

Alarming as it might sound, a course of colonic irrigation – or enemas – is a very good idea for any man over the age of about 35 who wants to keep his system functioning to the best of its abilities. By that time in life, especially if your eating habits haven't been that healthy, the chances are there will be a layer of built-up crud in your large intestine. This can restrict the absorption of nutrients, cause excess gas and bad breath, give you a perpetual bloated feeling and press on the bladder to limit its capacity and send you to the toilet more frequently (having to get up in the night is often caused by this condition). During an enema a tube is inserted in the anus and fluid is drained into the colon; it is kept there for a while then released under its own gravity into the toilet bowl. Just how much the average man needs during a week-long course of colonic irrigation becomes apparent as the treatment progresses. Each time, you will feel the fluid travelling further up your intestines and it will stay there a little bit longer. At the end of each enema the expelled material will be thicker, more continuous and eventually will resemble an impression of the intestine wall.

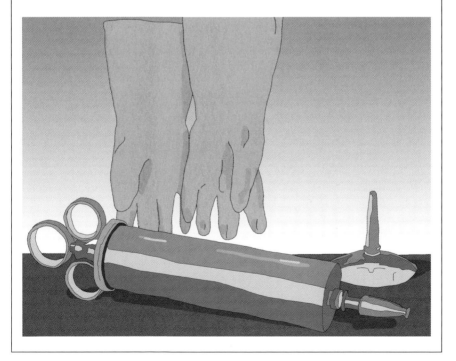

Sick sick sick

These are commonplace digestive system symptoms, and under most circumstances merely mean you've picked up a stomach bug. But the stomach is a pretty good healing machine, so if problems persist seek professional medical advice.

Vomiting

If you are suffering from simple food poisoning, this shouldn't last more than a couple of days.

Diarrhoea

Like vomiting, this is usually short-lived and most cases respond to commercially available remedies.

Stomach cramps

Could simply be indigestion or trapped wind, but if you are plagued with cramps for any length of time it might be irritable bowel syndrome.

Gnawing stomach pains

If they flare up sharply at times and are quietened down by eating or drinking milk, you could have an ulcer. Persistent pain might even signal the beginning of stomach cancer. But not always.

Blood in stools

Could be a bleeding ulcer or some other rupture of the stomach or intestine lining; this is also one of the first symptoms of colon cancer.

Constipation

If you've switched to a fibre-rich diet, drink loads of water and you still can't go, don't try chemical laxatives – they are never a good idea. Wait it out until it comes out.

Excess gas

Could be down to diet or poorly digested food; your doctor will probably recommend an enema.

FOOD POISONING

This is the most common and widespread form of gastroenteritis (see opposite), brought on by contaminated food introducing bacteria to the digestive system. There are nearly 50,000 cases of food poisoning reported in the UK each year, the most common being caused by salmonella, E-Coli and listeria bacteria. Contamination can result from food not being prepared or stored with proper attention to hygiene, or from food not being cooked properly, or from lack of personal hygiene on the part of the food handler. Depending on the severity of the contamination, the symptoms of food poisoning symptoms vary, but they usually include nausea and vomiting, sweating, dizziness and diarrhoea. On rare occasions, food poisoning requires hospitalisation. For less severe cases, the best treatment is rest, plenty of water and no solid food until the infection has passed.

The Irritable Bowel Self Help Group formed in 1987 and can be accessed on-line via www.ibsgroup.org. It claims that between 10 and 20 per cent of adults in America suffer from IBS. And they ain't just talking gas and hot air. They hold interactive chats on the site every Wednesday and Sunday.

IRRITABLE BOWEL SYNDROME (IBS)

This is more the name given to a collection of unexplained symptoms rather than an ailment in itself. Also known as spastic colon, the complaint is believed to be the result of involuntary muscle spasms in the large intestine leading to stomach cramps and bouts of diarrhoea and constipation. There is no real cure for IBS, although a high-fibre diet is believed to help relieve it, and the symptoms tend to come and go throughout a sufferer's life. The only good news is that men are much less likely to be affected than women.

GASTROENTERITIS

Montezuma's Revenge or Delhi Belly – this is the upset stomach you are liable to suffer from on holiday through bacterial or viral infections entering the stomach. Untreated water and contaminated food (see Food poisoning, left) are common causes. Dysentery, typhoid and cholera are severe forms of gastroenteritis. Rest, plenty of fluids, and a non-spicy diet are the best cures for mild gastroenteritis, but should symptoms persist it could be a serious infection and you should seek medical attention.

HAEMORRHOIDS

This is not really an ailment of the digestive system, but it occurs in the same general vicinity and is more than likely contributed to by digestive disorders. Occurring either internally or externally, they're one of life's more humorous conditions – for everybody, that is, except the sufferer.

They are swollen blood vessels in the anus that make sitting down or going to the toilet extremely painful. Haemorrhoids are often an inherited weakness – some people suffer with them their entire lives – but they can be caused through straining to pass faeces. (Women often get haemorrhoids through straining during childbirth.)

A high-fibre diet and drinking more water can help to make faeces softer and easier to pass, and may be enough to alleviate the problem. Otherwise, haemorrhoids are usually got rid of with over-the-counter creams or suppositories containing corticosteroids. If they persist, injections or minor surgical treatment may be necessary.

Intestinal outposts

Just beyond the stomach and intestines are a few organs that can cause you a good deal of trouble if they're not looked after.

THE LIVER

The liver is the biggest, heaviest organ in a man's body and is also one of the hardest working, given that it carries out about 5000 separate functions as part of the metabolic process. This organ is the body's chemical works, processing the nutrients brought in by the bloodstream and moving the results to the cells in the tissues and organs. The liver manufactures cholesterol from fats within food – everybody needs a degree of cholesterol for cell construction and creation of some hormones (see box, page 128). Bile is made in the liver from wastes in blood, before being stored in the gallbladder (see right) and fed into the small intestine to metabolise fats into usable form. Proteins produced in the liver help in the manufacture of plasma (the watery part of blood), and also form part of the immune system. The blood's coagulation factors begin life in the liver, as does globin, the active part of the red pigment haemoglobin that carries oxygen around the bloodstream. The liver converts surplus glucose (sugar) from food into glycogen, stores it until the body needs an energy boost, then converts it back to glucose and releases it into the system.

And perhaps most importantly, the liver breaks down the toxins in the blood, rendering them harmless.

THE PANCREAS

This large, elongated gland sits just behind the stomach and works in two main ways, aiding the digestive system and producing vital hormones. The pancreas produces the enzymes that break down fats, carbohydrates and proteins into usable form, and it does this by secreting them into the small intestine as digestive juices. It also produces the hormones insulin and glucagon and feeds them directly into the bloodstream, where they are vital for controlling the amount of sugar absorbed into the blood (see Diabetes, pages 142–47).

THE GALLBLADDER

Connected by ducts to the liver and the small intestine, the gallbladder is a small sac that stores bile (a digestive juice produced in the liver as a concentrate) and releases it into the small intestine as needed. Although the gallbladder is a handy reservoir, you could actually live without it. Sometimes the gallbladder has to be surgically removed following infection or because of recurring gallstones (see page 99), in which case the bile flows straight from the liver to the intestine.

The liver, pancreas and gallbladder

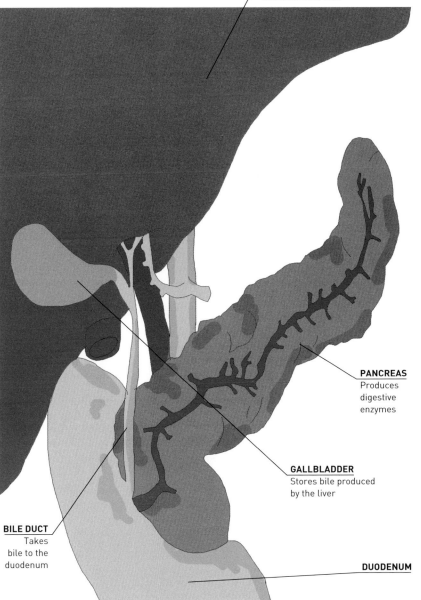

LIVER
Processes nutrients carried
in the bloodstream

PANCREAS
Produces
digestive
enzymes

GALLBLADDER
Stores bile produced
by the liver

BILE DUCT
Takes
bile to the
duodenum

DUODENUM

Feeling liverish?

As it's such a complicated organ, there's quite a lot that can go wrong with a liver – oh, and you shouldn't neglect your pancreas, either ...

DRINK-RELATED LIVER COMPLAINTS

The liver is a pretty difficult organ to kill, not least because coping with toxins is all in a day's work. Also, because it is so complex and vital to so much of the body's functioning, the liver has pretty good built-in defences, can regenerate itself and will continue to perform its functions even if half of it has been destroyed. But if you are determined to shut down your liver then the best way to do it is to drink excessively over a long period of time.

Even prolonged moderate drinking affects the liver, because it has to work so hard to process the toxins in the alcohol it hasn't got enough energy to do everything else properly, and fats will build up in it. But stop drinking for a while and this accumulation will be dispersed. Persistent drinking can lead to alcoholic hepatitis, which destroys cells within the liver but again, if you stop, the liver will right itself and regenerate. The big one is cirrhosis, for which there is no way back. Over 5000 people a year in the UK die from alcohol-related cirrhosis of the liver. This is what happens when the continued assault from the toxins in drink causes internal scarring and leaves liver cells too damaged to carry out their functions; so the liver packs up. A liver transplant is the only option under these circumstances, but the operation is very rarely carried out for such a self-inflicted condition. Stopping drinking before your liver actually stops working is the nearest thing to a cure for cirrhosis; although by this stage the liver cannot regenerate, its functioning will improve.

VIRAL HEPATITIS

Any inflammation of the liver is called hepatitis, and there are various causes. Viral hepatitis is caused by infection with several types of virus, classed as A, B, C, D or E. Hepatitis A can be spread through contaminated food or water in much the same way as food poisoning, and is the mildest form of infection. The most common causes of the B, C, and D infections are contaminated needles – intravenous drug users are particularly prone to viral hepatitis – contaminated blood from transfusion, or unprotected sex with a carrier of the disease. Hepatitis E is spread in a similar way to hepatitis A but is less common worldwide. Hepatitis symptoms are very similar to flu. The disease usually clears up by itself after a few weeks of rest and healthy eating.

PANCREATITIS

This is an inflammation of the pancreas brought on, usually, by alcohol abuse. It can also be a side effect of gallstones (see right), as they block the dispersal of the acidic juices produced in the pancreas, and the inflammation occasionally occurs as the result of viral hepatitis (see above). Pancreatitis may result in severe abdominal pain, swelling in the abdomen that is sore to the touch, nausea and fever. The disorder may clear up by itself after two or three days, unless it is the result of sustained alcohol abuse, in which case it is likely to persist for as long as the heavy drinking does. Severe or long-term pancreatitis can be dangerous, leading to permanent damage to the pancreas.

JAUNDICE

This is a symptom of various disorders and not a disease in itself. Jaundice is a yellowing of the whites of the eyes and, in Caucasians, a yellowing of the skin, which may be accompanied by very dark urine. It is caused by a high level in the bloodstream of the pigment bilirubin, which is normally filtered out of the liver as a component of bile. Jaundice is an indication of medical conditions that can include malaria, gallstones, liver malfunction or hepatitis. Anybody exhibiting signs of jaundice should seek urgent medical attention and assistance.

Gallstones

This condition is increasing in frequency in the developed world as diets change and obesity and cholesterol levels rise. Gallstones are tiny solids that are liable to form in the gallbladder when there is too much cholesterol in the chemical balance of the bile. These tiny particles can then collect more cholesterol and calcium from the bile and snowball into lumps as big as golf balls. In some instances, gallstones can block the bile duct and lead to inflammation of the gallbladder. They cause pain in the gut – usually during eating – and can be accompanied by fever and vomiting, possibly even jaundice. These symptoms are often confused with those of flu or some sort of viral infection, so if you are being investigated for ailments that could produce a similar effect it is important that you are examined for gallstones. Treatment for gallstones varies from medication that slowly dissolves the stones – this can take a year or more – to bombardment with shockwaves to shatter the stones, or surgery to remove the gallbladder.

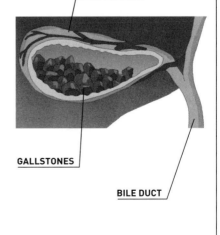

GALLBLADDER

GALLSTONES

BILE DUCT

Making the piss

The other waste disposal system in your body involves your kidneys and bladder, which handle the liquids.

The kidneys are among the most under-appreciated organs in a man's body, yet they are two of the hardest working. For instance, if you go out on the lash then you'll talk a lot about what your liver has to cope with, but spare a thought for your kidneys. They have to deal with those nine additional beers and work out what to get rid of (most of it) and what should be kept to make the body function more efficiently (not much of it). But then processing the fall-out from nine pints of beer isn't, relatively speaking, that much when you consider that the average man's kidneys deal with nearly 40 times that quantity of fluid every day. That's how much blood gets pumped through them to be filtered and returned to use.

The kidneys are situated at the very back of the abdominal cavity, one on either side of the spine. One of their biggest jobs is to regulate the body's fluid levels and to adjust the balance of toxins, acids and certain hormones that the fluid contains. The

Diabetics and their kidneys

Because of the potential for kidney damage as the result of high levels of blood sugar, 25 per cent of all diabetics suffer from some sort of kidney complaint, although it is usually later in life. It is a cumulative process and there may be many years between someone being diagnosed as diabetic and suffering kidney damage. If you are diabetic you should have regular urine tests – at least twice a year – to monitor your kidney function and to check that your blood sugar levels remain below 8 mmol/l. Diabetics also need to be very careful to keep their kidneys working properly because of the role the organs play in regulating blood pressure.

Hippocrates, the world's first proper doctor, used to prescribe drinking urine to heal yourself. However, that was more than 2000 years ago, and some things have changed a bit since then. (Don't try it.)

The kidneys

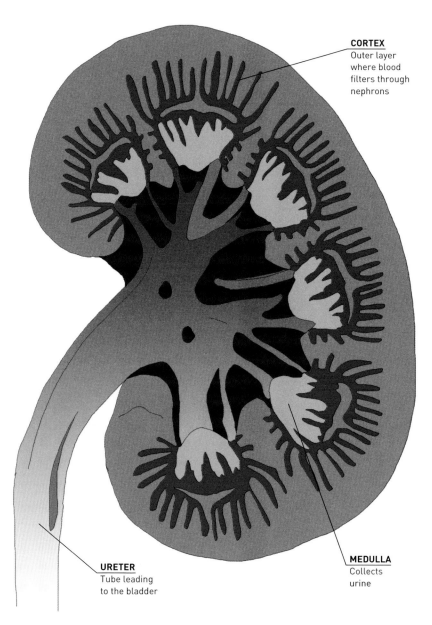

CORTEX
Outer layer where blood filters through nephrons

MEDULLA
Collects urine

URETER
Tube leading to the bladder

kidneys also stimulate red blood cell production by bone marrow and, by controlling the volume of blood, have a great deal of responsibility for blood pressure. Despite this heavy workload, just one working kidney can keep the body functioning normally.

Roughly 150 litres (260 pints) of blood per day flow through the kidneys from the heart via the renal artery, which branches directly from the aorta. Inside the kidneys, blood is filtered and processed. The waste products from metabolic activity, muscle effort and the digestive system are flushed away with excess water and electrolytes (minerals) and taken to the bladder to be passed as urine. A great many substances in the blood are useful to the body, though, so the kidneys sort these out and make sure they go back into the bloodstream.

In each kidney the filtering is done by approximately a million tiny units called nephrons that are situated in the outer part of the kidney, the cortex. As blood flows through the nephrons every extra element is removed from it, and what is to be taken back into the system and what is to be got rid of are separated. The waste is converted into urine and drains away into the ureters, tubes that run from the kidneys to the

Kidney stones

It's not unusual for crystals or tiny solids to occur in the kidneys as a result of chemicals and minerals being filtered out of the bloodstream. Normally, these pass out of the body unnoticed when you urinate. Occasionally, however, the materials build up to form solid masses large enough to cause considerable discomfort or even blockage in the urinary tract. Kidney stones are far more common in men than women, particularly in men in their twenties and thirties; and, for unknown reasons, they are far more common in Caucasians than any other ethnic group. The symptoms of kidney stones are:

Shooting pains in your lower back and side. |

Blood in your urine. |

Hot and cold sweats, vomiting, fever and fatigue (the signs of kidney stones are often confused with flu). |

Constant desire to urinate, even though when you try you can't, or you have just been. |

Burning sensation during urination. |

Urinary tract infections

These are fairly uncommon in men, because the length of the male urethra means that infection from outside is unlikely to get very far into the urinary system. However, infection from within is possible, either from bacteria seeping in from the digestive system or originating in stagnant urine in the bladder, or being carried into the kidneys via the bloodstream. Kidney stones (see box on left) or an enlarged prostate gland can block the excretion of wastes, allowing bacteria to multiply. Diabetics are particularly prone to kidney and bladder infections. Any infection of the urinary system should be treated as soon as possible, as it can spread and cause kidney damage. The early warning signs are:

Frequent urination

This can result in dehydration if you are not drinking enough to make up for the loss of fluid.

Painful urination

Internal burning sensations may be felt during urination and an itching at the opening of your penis afterwards.

Unusual-looking urine

Cloudy, dark brown, reddish, milky ... anything out of the ordinary over a sustained period of time could indicate an infection.

Being unable to urinate or slowing in mid-stream

You may feel you have a full bladder but can't empty it properly.

Research published in 2004 stated that there was a definite link between people with even mild kidney disease and coronary disease. Mild kidney dysfunction raised the chances of death by 20 per cent. More severe kidney disease increased the risk of death sixfold. (New England Journal of Medicine)

Dialysis

If, for whatever reason, the kidneys pack up and a transplant isn't immediately available, toxins can build to dangerous levels within the body. This means that the kidneys' functions have to be fulfilled by artificial means – dialysis. Treatment can be short term, while a damaged kidney awaits repair, or long term because whatever is wrong with the kidneys is uncurable. There are two main methods: one, haemodialysis, purifies the blood through an artificial kidney and the other, peritoneal dialysis, uses a membrane in the abdomen as a substitute filter.

HAEMODIALYSIS

For this treatment, the patient is attached to an artificial kidney (a kidney machine) through tubes inserted into blood vessels. The patient's blood flows into the machine where it is purified as it passes through a series of membranes, and the clean blood is then returned to the body. This procedure, which can last up to six hours, usually takes place at specialised outpatients' centres and needs be done two or three times a week.

PERITONEAL DIALYSIS

This type of dialysis uses a membrane in the patient's abdominal cavity, known as the peritoneum, as a blood filter. A fluid called dialysate is dripped into the cavity of the abdomen, where it is left for several hours to collect wastes and excess water that pass into it from the blood vessels in the peritoneum. The dialysate, carrying the potential toxins, is then drained out through a catheter surgically inserted into the abdomen through the skin. Fresh dialysate is emptied into the abdomen to repeat the cycle. Patients are taught how to perform peritoneal dialysis themselves at home and can get on with their normal lives in between the infusion and draining procedures.

bladder. In the inner part of the kidney, which is called the medulla, the good stuff that was removed is reabsorbed back into the bloodstream and carried back into the system via the renal vein.

The bladder is a hollow, balloon-like organ with powerful muscles that control the outlet to the urethra in the penis. It fills as the kidneys send urine in short bursts and its elastic walls expand to store the urine until the brain receives signals that the bladder is full. Urine runs into the bladder more or less continuously, because if it was allowed to hang around in the ureters it would quickly cause infection. Because the muscles at the bladder's outlet valve are under the control of the brain, it is possible to consciously ignore the desire to urinate, but that is also why the sound of running water will make you want to go.

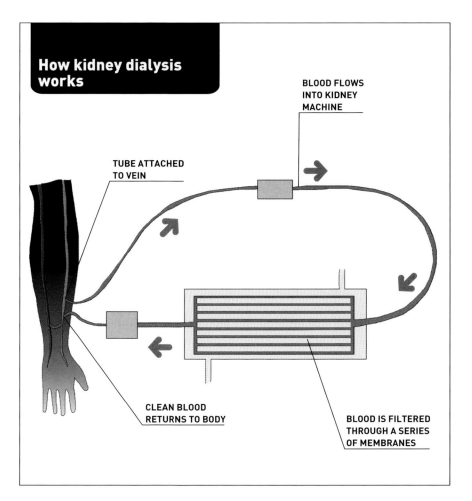

How kidney dialysis works

BLOOD FLOWS INTO KIDNEY MACHINE

TUBE ATTACHED TO VEIN

CLEAN BLOOD RETURNS TO BODY

BLOOD IS FILTERED THROUGH A SERIES OF MEMBRANES

You are what you eat

Diet is the quickest and easiest way for a man to start looking after his health, yet as we progress into the 21st-century healthy eating is becoming increasingly neglected.

A balanced diet is the starting point for good living. Without it, no matter what other precautions or actions you might take, you will stand a much smaller chance of living a healthy life. Your chances of a full life are affected, too, as it is through eating we take on board the basic materials that supply energy to our muscles and build and repair cells for growth and healing. Diet is an integral part of medicine both as prevention and cure. Correcting a bad diet can prevent the likelihood of such conditions as heart disease, osteoporosis (brittle bones) or diabetes, while changing a diet by introducing new elements or cutting out old ones can greatly assist recovery from illness or the combating of bacteria.

A healthy diet is one that balances the five major food groups: cereals/grains/rice; fruit and vegetables; plant protein; animal protein; and dairy products. This provides something from each category but isn't overloaded with one thing at the expense of another. As well as specific vitamins and minerals (see pages 112–17) what you are looking for in your diet are carbohydrates for

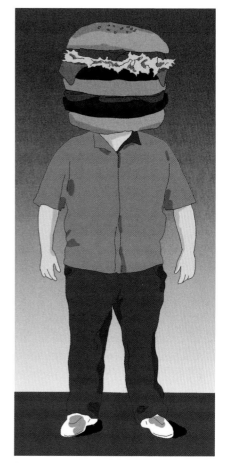

When you look in a mirror, is this what you see? If your name is Mr Burgerhead, then that's fine.

Instant action

If your diet is typically male – not very good and probably not getting any better – here are five things to remember if you want to conquer the basics of healthy eating.

LESS SUGAR

Refined sugar, either in drinks or in cakes and confectionery, means empty calories so although you are taking on board energy no other nutrients are coming in with it. And that's without considering the tooth decay end of the equation. Cutting out sugar is one of the best ways to rebalance your diet, but watch out for it as a 'hidden' ingredient in many processed foods.

MORE FIBRE

This not only prevents constipation, but helps to get fats and sugar into the bloodstream in controlled amounts, preventing spikes and crashes in blood sugar levels. Fruit, vegetables, whole grains, cereal and pulses are good sources of fibre.

LESS SALT

Salt can lead to high blood pressure as once in the system it attracts water, so waste fluids stay in the body and the volume of your blood increases. Be very careful of processed foods and prepared meat products as these usually contain much more salt than is strictly good for you.

MORE WATER

It keeps things flowing, stops you eating too much and helps your body make more efficient use of many of the vitamins and minerals provided by other foods.

LESS FAT

Although some fat is good for you (see page 110), too much, especially of the saturated fats, can lead to weight gain, high blood pressure, type 2 diabetes and an increased chance of heart disease. Cut down on animal fats and dairy products, use more olive oil or vegetable oils and check processed food labels carefully for trans fats, a potentially deadly ingredient.

energy; protein for maintenance and growth of muscle, bone and body tissue; and fat for vitamins and hormone production. The ideal diet for maximum efficiency is high in fibre but low in fat and sugar. This means whole grains, pulses and cereals should figure prominently, fruit and vegetables should outweigh meat and dairy foods, and fat for fat's sake (butter and cooking oil, for instance) and sugar should feature as little as possible.

You don't have to eat boringly to eat healthily, but you might have to apply some greater thought. However, the plus side is that when you start fully exploring the healthy eating possibilities you will surprise

Water! water!

Although they have got much better about it over the last few years, men in general still don't drink nearly enough water. Water keeps everything moving through your system with a minimum of fuss and constantly replenishes your body's water levels, which make up roughly 60 to 70 per cent of your body weight. It's worth remembering that often when you think you feel hungry you are in fact thirsty, and thirst is a warning that your body's water levels have dipped far too low. Don't try to quench your thirst with sugary soft drinks, fruit juice or beer as these don't give your body the water it needs and will leave you still feeling thirsty.

How much water you need varies according to factors such as physical exertion – the more active you are, the more you should drink. You should also drink more if the temperature is rising or you are sweating; and if you have an illness such as diarrhoea that depletes your body's fluid levels, you need to up your water intake.

Under normal circumstances, though, an average healthy man should be drinking 2 litres (3½ pints) of water a day. And remember that it is particularly important to have a drink first thing in the morning, as a night's sleep leaves you dehydrated.

It also helps to clear a hangover faster than supposed 'cures'.

yourself with how fabulous the menu can taste. Honest.

CARBOHYDRATES

Carbs, which come from plants and comprise fibre, starch and sugars, are our main source of dietary energy. Ideally, carbohydrates should make up just over half of your calorific intake. There are two main types of carbohydrates and they both work for you in different ways. They are known as simple carbohydrates and complex carbohydrates. The former, also called simple sugars, provide a calorific value but nothing else – empty calories is what they are often called. Simple carbs are in refined sugar, maple syrup, corn syrup, honey or the natural

sugars that occur in fresh fruit. They fill you up without providing any nutritional value and so leave you feeling hungry again, leading to overeating and weight gain. Also, as simple carbs are absorbed into the system so quickly they cause a 'sugar rush' followed by an energy crash. Complex carbs are starches or fibre and are taken into the system much more slowly, thus providing regular, long-term energy. They are nutrient-rich and the fibre aids digestion and prevents constipation. Complex carbohydrates are found in whole grains, some fruit and vegetables (potatoes are rich in complex carbs), pulses and cereals. Wholewheat pasta, brown rice or wholemeal bread are good sources of complex carbohydrates.

What about eating in restaurants?

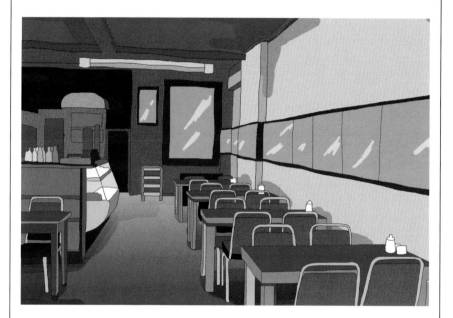

That's simple. Nobody is suggesting you should give up eating out; simply follow the same food guidelines as you would at home. Make sensible choices from the menu, and if in doubt ask the waiter – if the staff of a restaurant are reluctant to tell you what's in a particular dish then it's probably not a good idea to be eating there. Also, don't be scared to ask for something prepared in a particular way, for instance, with no butter or no salt; most good restaurants will only be too happy to oblige. If your favourite restaurant offers no healthy options then make dining there just an occasional treat.

PROTEIN

Protein builds the body's tissues and repairs damages. It is made up of 21 different amino acids, nine of which cannot be produced internally and therefore have to come from the food we eat. There are two types of protein: animal protein, which comes from meat, dairy products, eggs and poultry; and vegetable protein, found in cereals, pulses, rice and nuts. Animal proteins are richer in amino acids and therefore offer a more reliable source of nourishment, but it is possible for vegans to obtain all the protein they need from combination of beans, whole rice and nuts. In modern times people, especially men, tend to eat much more protein than they need – a 170-gram (6-oz) serving of meat or chicken or a half a litre (one pint) of milk or three eggs a day would be ample. Although excess protein won't necessarily do any harm it might be eaten to the exclusion of foods that provide other important nutrients.

FATS

The good news is that not all fat is bad for you. Although fats contribute to your cholesterol levels, not all cholesterol will kill you and some even goes a long way to keeping you alive (see box, page 128). It will be of considerable benefit to you to recognise the good, the bad and the deadly when it comes to sorting out your eating plan. There are three main types of fats: monounsaturated, polyunsaturated and saturated.

Monounsaturated fats are, essentially, one of the good guys. They lower all blood cholesterol levels, but decrease the dangerous cholesterol in greater amounts, so in effect working to increase the supply of 'good' cholesterol that you do need. Monounsaturates are found in vegetable oils – notably olive oil – fish, seafood and avocados. Polyunsaturated fats also reduce all cholesterol proportionately and contribute greatly to keeping down the levels of harmful cholesterol. Vegetable oils are good sources of polyunsaturated fats, olive oil in particular, and so are soya beans and oily fish. Polyunsaturates are rich in chemicals known as essential fatty acids, which are a very good idea as they reduce high blood pressure by thinning the blood and they also diminish the likelihood of clotting, therefore considerably cutting down the risk of heart disease. Omega-3 and omega-6 are the most common essential fatty acids and are found in abundance in oily fish such as salmon, mackerel or sardines.

Saturated fats raise all cholesterol levels in your body and, in particular, they boost levels of the dangerous stuff. The main

Lard is clarified pig fat. One tablespoon of lard contains 116 calories, 13 grams of fat and 12 mg of cholesterol.

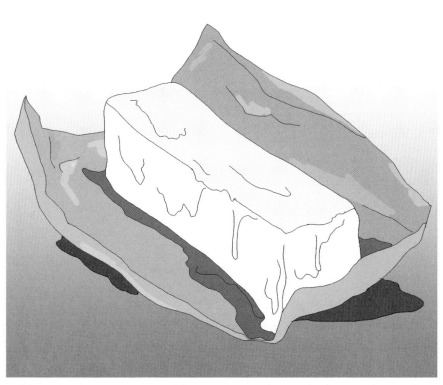

Lard. Homer loves it and mass-produced chips and various crap foods use it because it's cheap. But it's very, very bad for you. So you can wash with it, uses it as a sexual aid but never, ever eat it.

sources of saturated fats are animal rather than vegetable fats, with red meat, most dairy products, bacon and lard being particularly popular.

There are other types of fats, known as trans fats or hydrogenated fats, that are similar to saturated fats. These are totally manmade and are found in processed food. Basically, trans fats in excess can kill you. They will raise your 'bad' cholesterol to stratospheric levels and do nothing at all helpful for your system. Watch out for them by checking food labels. The clue is 'partially hydrogenised oils' – if that's what it says on the label then the product contains trans fats.

It isn't necessary to completely cut fat out of your healthy eating plan – just as well, given that old cook's saying 'the flavour is in the fat' – but you need to pay a bit more attention to how you consume it. Switch to unsaturated fats wherever possible; shallow fry food instead of deep frying it or, better still, use another method such as grilling; change to low fat milk and cheese; stop using butter and start buying olive oil spread; and avoid trans fats altogether.

The A to K of vitamins

Unless you are able to eat totally organically, or can grow all your own food, the chances are your diet isn't doing all it can for you. And the more processed or factory-farmed foods you eat the more your diet could be actively working against you. As modern-day life requires increasing amounts of energy and the stress factors pile up, it becomes ever more vital to get the nutrients we need to function efficiently and healthily. Yet eating often falls victim to lifestyle and with lack of time or the pressure of social obligations basic nutrition gets pushed to one side. Astonishingly, in the developed world, more and more incidences of malnutrition – especially among young, single men – are showing up when people are being investigated for health complaints.

The simple truth is we have to take on board certain vitamins and minerals and carbohydrates and proteins in order for our bodies to work, and today that might be in supplement form as much as through food. But in order to stay healthy and nourished in a high-speed world, you first have to understand fully what does what and what, exactly, you need.

WHAT THEY DO, WHY YOU NEED THEM AND WHERE TO FIND THEM

VITAMIN A
What it does: Promotes growth and is essential for bones, teeth, eyesight and for healthy, clear skin.
If you don't get enough: Poor eyesight in anything less than bright light, dry scratchy

Vitamin B complex

Not complex at all really. In fact, it's pretty straightforward! Vitamin B complex is a combination of vitamins B1, B2, B3 (niacin), B6, B12, pantothenic acid, biotin and folic acid. It is available in tablet form, and is believed to be the best way to take the B vitamin family as a supplement, because you need such small amounts of some of them.

eyes, skin problems such as boils and acne.
Found in: Liver, fish oils, dairy foods, tomatoes, green vegetables, oranges.

VITAMIN B1 (thiamin)
What it does: Helps to convert carbohydrates into energy, maintains and repairs the nervous system.
If you don't get enough: Tiredness, poor muscle function, lack of appetite.
Found in: Wheatgerm, whole grains, brown rice, nuts, beans, eggs, liver.

VITAMIN B2 (riboflavin)
What it does: Assists in breaking down food to release energy, repairs body tissues, maintains lubricating mucus in upper respiratory system, assists in adrenaline production.

If you don't get enough: Chapped lips and mouth sores.
Found in: Brewer's yeast, liver, eggs, dairy foods, leafy vegetables, whole grains.

VITAMIN B3 (niacin)
What it does: Assists in the metabolisation of carbohydrates and fats, helps to maintain the nervous system, produces sex hormones, promotes healthy skin.
If you don't get enough: Dryness and soreness of the mouth, low sex drive, dry skin.
Found in: Liver, poultry, nuts, beans.

VITAMIN B6 (pyridoxine)
What it does: Assists in the breakdown of foods to release energy, manufactures red blood cells, regulates the nervous system, essential for healthy skin.

If you don't get enough: Anaemia, skin complaints, irritability, maybe even depression.
Found in: Liver, whole grains, bananas, potatoes, fish.

VITAMIN B12
What it does: Produces red blood cells in bone marrow, promotes growth by the formation of genetic materials, assists with the functioning of the nervous system.
If you don't get enough: Anaemia, possibly pins and needles in the extremities.
Found in: Liver, kidneys, beef, pork, chicken, eggs, dairy foods.

BIOTIN (vitamin H, but usually grouped with the B vitamins)
What it does: Manufactures new cells, assists with the removal of waste products

RDA (recommended daily allowances)

mg = milligrams; mcg = micrograms

VITAMIN	Man in his 20s	In his 30s	In his 40s	Over 50
A	1000 mg	1000 mg	1000 mg	1000 mg
B1 (thiamine)	1.5 mg	1.4 mg	1.4 mg	1.2 mg
B3 (niacin)	19 mg	18 mg	17 mg	16 mg
B12	3.0 mcg	3.0 mcg	3.0 mcg	3.0 mcg
Folic acid	400 mcg	400 mcg	400 mcg	400 mcg
B2 (riboflavin)	1.7 mg	1.6 mg	1.5 mg	1.4 mg
C	60 mg	60 mg	60 mg	60 mg
D	10 mcg	7.5 mcg	5.0 mcg	5.0 mcg
E	10 mg	10 mg	10 mg	10 mg

following the metabolisation of food.
If you don't get enough: Tiredness, hair loss, anaemia, lack of appetite.
Found in: Liver, beans, nuts, bananas, grapefruit.

PANTOTHENIC ACID (a B vitamin)
What it does: Assists in the metabolisation of carbohydrates and fats, helps other vitamins get into the system, produces sex hormones, aids the functioning of the nervous system.
If you don't get enough: Abdominal pains, headaches, fatigue, low sex drive.
Found in: Vegetables, cereal, nuts, liver.

FOLIC ACID
What it does: Produces red blood cells, assists in the functioning of the nervous system, promotes growth by the manufacture of cells.
If you don't get enough: Anaemia, stunted growth in children.
Found in: Leafy green vegetables, nuts, egg yolk, liver, whole grains.

VITAMIN C
What it does: Maintains healthy bones, teeth, gums and blood vessels, assists the immune system, helps the body to absorb iron, boosts the adrenal glands.

If you don't get enough: Fatigue, loose teeth, bleeding and swollen gums, anaemia.
Found in: Leafy green vegetables, citrus fruits, blackcurrants, kiwi fruits, strawberries, green peppers.

VITAMIN D
What it does: Regulates calcium levels in the body, vital for growth and maintenance of bones and teeth.
If you don't get enough: Fragile bones, liver and kidney disorders.
Found in: Fish oils, liver, eggs.

VITAMIN E
What it does: Promotes healthy cell structure, destroys free radicals (harmful molecules), protects red blood cells, guards lungs against pollution damage.
If you don't get enough: Anaemia due to the destruction of red blood cells.
Found in: Leafy green vegetables, vegetable oils, nuts, lean meat, egg yolk.

VITAMIN K
What it does: Helps the blood to clot.
If you don't get enough: Nose bleeds, bleeding gums, slow healing of cuts, possibly intestinal bleeding.
Found in: Leafy green vegetables, vegetable oils, egg yolk, cheese.

Supplementary benefit

The global vitamin supplement industry is worth over $20 billion per year, yet a fierce debate is going on as to whether this is money well spent or wasted. While the manufacturers of vitamin pills and powders maintain that our bodies need all the help they can get, an opposing school of thought has it that anybody who maintains a healthy and balanced diet has no need for supplements. And both sides are right. In theory, we should get all the nutrients we need from the food we eat but, in reality, fewer and fewer people do these days. As mentioned earlier, incidences of malnutrition in this country are rising dramatically.

The main reason for poor nutrition is the increased consumption of processed and convenience foods, as most of the ingredients' intrinsic goodness frequently gets lost in the processing. Then the propagation of fruit and vegetables to look better and last longer in the supermarkets has further contributed to the vitamin-shaped hole in so many diets, because changing anything in the food's natural balance risks destroying its nutritional value. Careless cooking doesn't help either; many vegetables' nutritional elements are water-soluble and destroyed by boiling. Also, if you eat in restaurants and canteens, it's worth remembering that keeping food on a hot plate for a quarter of an hour after cooking destroys roughly 25 per cent of its vitamin content;

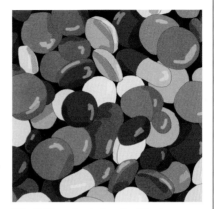

Pills, thrills and no belly ache. Vitamins are the kind of pills that you should be popping.

letting it stand for over an hour will kill off up to 75 per cent. The result of all this is that people are eating more to make up for the relative lack of nourishment per serving of food.

Of course, not everybody has time or the means to buy produce direct from an organic farm, then cook each meal at home to strict guidelines and eat it immediately. Many people – notably young men – rely on takeaways, eating out and convenience food to fit in with their busy lives, and therefore ought to be taking vitamin supplements to make sure they get what they need despite what they eat. A word of warning, though, if you buy multi-vitamin tablets, read the labels carefully to make sure they will deliver the recommended daily allowances of what you need (see page 113).

Mineral wealth

Minerals are chemicals that your body needs to function properly. Unlike vitamins, which occur naturally in the foods we eat, minerals are absorbed into food from external sources – the water, the soil or further along the food chain, when animals have eaten plants containing certain minerals. Because we need many minerals only in microscopic amounts, it is easier to take in an excess (which may be harmful) than to incur a deficiency. There are 20 different minerals that the body needs in varying amounts; those listed below are the seven most important.

CALCIUM
What it does: Makes the muscles work (more than any other mineral), makes cells function, assists with blood clotting and is the main ingredient of bones and teeth.
If you don't get enough: Brittle bones (osteoporosis) or restricted growth in

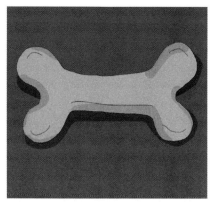

Dog biscuits. Full of calcium, good for teeth and will give you a shiny coat.

children, malfunctioning of muscles and nerve endings.
Too much can: Cause constipation or, eventually, kidney stones.
Found in: Dairy foods, eggs, fish (especially ones like sardines with edible bones), leafy green vegetables.
Deficiency can be caused by: Calcium deficiency is almost unheard of, as the body has vast reserves in the bones.
Recommended daily allowance: 700 mg

CHROMIUM
What it does: Promotes efficient working of many of the enzymes that keep the body functioning.
If you don't get enough: Deficiency is virtually unknown, as you need such tiny amounts of chromium.
Too much can: Poison you, but you'd need quite a lot. Prolonged exposure to chromium fumes can lead to lung cancer, though.
Found in: Red meat, dairy, green vegetables.
Recommended daily allowance: 500mcg

IRON
What it does: Essential for getting oxygen into red blood cells and carrying oxygen to the muscles.
If you don't get enough: Anaemia.
Too much can: Cause abdominal pain and constipation.
Found in: Leafy green vegetables, nuts, liver, whole grains, meat, fish.
Deficiency can be caused by: Heavy blood loss, or a diet devoid of fresh fruit and vegetables.
Recommended daily allowance: 8.75 mg

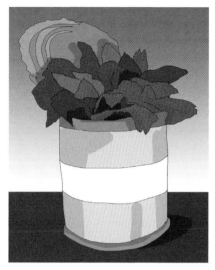

Good grief! Red spinach! What would Popeye have made of it? Oh, he was colour blind.

If you don't get enough: Fatigue, sleepiness, irregular heartbeat.
Too much can: Cause heartbeat irregularities, pins and needles.
Found in: Leafy green vegetables, bananas, oranges, lean meat.
Deficiency can be caused by: Gastroenteritis, diarrhoea or vomiting.
Recommended daily allowance: 3.5mg

SODIUM

What it does: Maintains your body's water levels, keeps the heartbeat regular, assists in muscle movement.
If you don't get enough: Cramp, dizziness, muscle weakness.
Too much can: Lead to high blood pressure, heart disease, water retention.
Found in: Nearly all food naturally contains some sodium; also table salt and cheese. Much processed food and snack food contains a worryingly high degree of salt.
Deficiency can be caused by: Profuse and prolonged sweating, diarrhoea or vomiting.
Recommended daily allowance: 1.6g

MAGNESIUM

What it does: Essential for the formation and maintenance of bones and teeth, for muscle function and a healthy nervous system.
If you don't get enough: Possibility of kidney stones; mental disturbances such as restlessness and depression.
Too much can: Cause nausea, vomiting, fatigue and muscle weakness. Prolonged excess can lead to heart disorders.
Found in: Nuts, whole grains, dairy foods, soya beans, fish.
Deficiency can be caused by: Kidney disease or a digestive disorder that blocks its absorption.
Recommended daily allowance: 300mg

POTASSIUM

What it does: Keeps the heartbeat regular, assists with muscle movement, regulates water levels in the body.

ZINC

What it does: Assists the functioning of the prostate gland, heals wounds, promotes effective insulin usage, aids sperm production, boosts circulation.
If you don't get enough: Loss of appetite, loss of hair.
Too much can: Cause abdominal pains, vomiting, fatigue.
Found in: Whole grains, seafood, lean meat.
Deficiency can be caused by: Sickle cell anaemia or the recovery from major injury such as a burn.
Recommended daily allowance: 9.5mg

Naturally, Jackson

Remarkably, in the face of medical advancements, natural remedies are increasing in popularity. These are a few that are recommended specifically for men's problems. (Remember, if you are taking any conventional medicines it may not be safe to use alternative remedies at the same time – always ask your doctor for advice.)

IMPOTENCE

Guta kola: This is a herb from Australia and the South Pacific. Taken as an infusion or as capsules, guta kola can increase blood flow to maintain erections longer and with less strain on the heart. It also assists in the healing of wounds and maintaining of nerve endings.

Bilberries: Powerful and effective all-round circulation boosters, bilberries strengthen the capillaries to allow a stronger blood flow without risk of the vessels rupturing.

Fo ti root: Used in Chinese herbalism as a specific cure for impotence, it is thought be another all-round circulation booster.

Saw palmetto berry: Among other properties this plant from southern Florida increases blood flow to the penis.

Suma: A Brazilian herb that is very similar in action to ginseng (see box, right) in as much as it acts as a general tonic. However, in South America suma is held in particular regard for its effects on impotence. It is taken in capsule form.

Damiana leaf: A considerable aphrodisiac that, by increasing sexual desire, will usually increase the ability to function.

Licorice root: Raises sexual performance and desire across the board but, be warned, it is also a pretty powerful natural laxative.

PREMATURE EJACULATION

Nutmeg: Either taken as a suspension in warm water or milk, or in capsule form, nutmeg has long been valued for its calming effect, which helps to slow the system down and prolong the period before ejaculation.

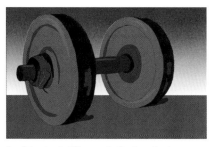

Don't be dumb, lift some bells. Exercise is, naturally, good for you. And gives you muscles.

A little something extra

Among the readily available natural remedies you need to keep yourself fit and healthy, there are three real high performers that will give you a considerable all-round boost. All perfectly legal, honest, officer. They are the three Gs: garlic, ginkgo and ginseng.

GARLIC

We've talked about the joys of garlic elsewhere (see page 49). It has many uses and is one of the most widely purchased health supplements in the world. Because garlic lowers blood pressure and keeps cholesterol levels down it is particularly useful in combating heart disease. But it also boosts the immune system as it is a natural antibiotic and fights invading bacteria – garlic is very good for AIDS sufferers, whose natural resistance is lowered. It functions as a glandular tonic, too, and has been shown to boost libido and improve sexual performance. Also, as garlic helps the whole digestive system work better it greatly assists in the metabolising of nutrients in other food.

GINKGO

This is an extract from the maidenhair tree (Ginkgo biloba), the best-selling herbal medicine in continental Europe. It is great for sharpening mental concentration and improving clarity of thought in general because it increases the supply of blood, and therefore oxygen, to the brain. Ginkgo improves circulation all around the body by strengthening the capillaries that carry blood to the tissues, meaning that they can safely carry more blood and deliver more oxygen. This has a particular impact in the brain and in the eyes, which are supplied by far more capillaries than elsewhere in the body. For the penis and its need for a frequently increased blood supply, ginkgo is an effective weapon against impotency or other erectile dysfunction. Gingko is favoured by the elderly, too, and is used to treat senile dementia, headaches and degenerative eye disorders.

GINSENG

One of the mainstays of Chinese herbal medicine, ginseng root has been recommended for men for centuries – indeed, in Chinese its original name, jen sen, means 'man root'. It is used as a general tonic because it contains substances called saponins, or ginsenosides, which are natural stress relievers as they reduce blood pressure and prevent blood sugar surges. By slowing the system down, saponins aid concentration and alertness, and promote clearheaded thinking by reducing the likelihood of panic attacks or adrenaline surges. Ginseng is also proven to be an energy booster, increasing stamina and aiding sexual performance by raising male hormone levels – as the Chinese see it, increasing the body's life-flow.

TESTOSTERONE BOOSTING

Saw palmetto berry: A reliable testosterone raiser, saw palmetto increases sex drive and, by acting as a mild aphrodisiac, sexual desire.

Sarsaparilla root: This stimulates the production of testosterone and also works to purify the blood and raise stamina.

INFERTILITY

Zinc: In recent tests, a majority of patients with a low sperm count were found to have low levels of zinc, although in all cases increased zinc did not automatically raise the sperm count.

L-carnitine: This is an amino acid that increases sperm mobility (increasing the likelihood of sperm reaching the egg) and potency.

Vitamin C: Increases sperm mobility.

Vitamin E: Raises sperms' potency levels, increasing the chances of fertilisation.

BALDNESS

Nothing has been proven to prevent or even slow down male pattern baldness, but turmeric taken as a suspension in fruit juice will keep existing hair thick and healthy and maintain its volume.

PROSTATE PROBLEMS

Saw palmetto berry: This is acknowledged worldwide for preventing enlargement of the prostate gland as it blocks the enzyme that transforms testosterone into dihydrotestosterone, which is what swells the gland.

Pygeum: Made from tree bark, this works in much the same way as saw palmetto berry.

Zinc: This not only helps to prevent prostate enlargement but can reduce existing swelling.

Evening primrose oil: Will reduce swelling in the prostate gland by producing the anti-inflammatory prostaglandins.

Licorice root: Believed to prevent the conditions in which prostate cancer can occur.

ANXIETY AND DEPRESSION

St John's wort: A widely recognised mood enhancer, this herb needs to be used over a period of time, as it takes about 30 days to fully get into your system. It has the unfortunate side effect of truly unbearable farts. (Consult your doctor before taking.)

Nutmeg: An accepted sedative, nutmeg helps you to sleep and improves the quality of sleep, which can greatly reduce anxiety.

Chamomile: Taken as a tea or infusion, this is soothing and relaxing – ideal for preventing anxiety attacks or maintaining clear headedness.

Vitamin B complex: These vitamins enhance the brain's neurotransmitters, or messengers, meaning that you think better and gain more control of your life.

Every healthy kitchen needs ...

If you're going to change your eating habits from fry-ups and takeaways to something that actually keeps you alive and kicking, the chances are your kitchen will need a bit of an overhaul. While there's no limit to what you can spend turning your cooking area into a centre for culinary excellence, there are a few things you'll need to start off with, just to make that healthy eating plan far more accessible.

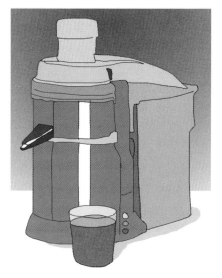

JUICER

It is widely accepted that carton juice is more or less worthless as regards nutritional value, so the only way to ensure you get the vitamin power you need is to drink juice straight from the fruit. Or, at least, you should drink it as soon after it's extracted as possible (fruit juice progressively loses its vitamin content once exposed to the atmosphere) and the only way to do this is to squeeze it yourself. Citrus presses or lemon squeezers are a good start. However, if you are drinking the amount of juice you ought to be it's worth investing in a electric squeezer, which is big enough to handle things like grapefruit. The next stage up is a juice extractor, into which you can feed any fruit you want, from apples to pineapples to root ginger to kiwis to oranges to melons, and create some truly fabulous and magnificently healthy concoctions.

Did you know that dandelion root contains insulin, which lowers blood sugar in diabetics? Dandelion is a great additive to most fruit smoothies. So get picking and juicing.

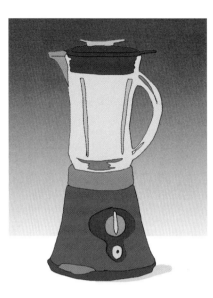

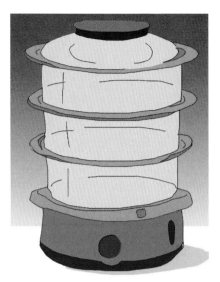

STEAMER

Steaming is by far the best method of cooking fresh vegetables without jeopardising their nutritional value. A steamer cooks all sorts of vegetables so quickly, and without immersing them in water, that any water-soluble vitamins (vitamins B and C) stand the greatest chance of surviving. Also, due to the speed of this process, cooked veg is far less likely to go limp and lose its colour or flavour – plus it's virtually impossible to put a lot of salt on to vegetables in a steamer.

BLENDER

Vegetable puree soups and protein fruit shakes should be part of every man's healthy eating plan, and the easiest way to make them is with a blender. Also, if you get a blender with a chopping attachment it will be perfect for grinding up nuts or finely chopping the herbs you'll be using in your cooking.

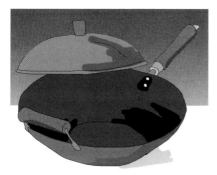

delicious smells, and you can set the timer so that you wake up in the morning to the freshest, nicest bread you've ever tasted. It's the one way to make sure the bread you eat contains nothing but healthy ingredients and it offers scope for a huge range of alternatives such as fruit bread, olive bread, walnut bread, garlic bread ...

WOK

Stir-frying vegetables and meat in a wok is a far healthier way of cooking than frying or boiling as you'll use far less fat and no water, thus vitamins are less likely to dissolve (vitamins A, D, E and K are fat soluble). Also, stir-frying tends to cook food quicker, retaining taste and texture, and it is possible to toss together some brilliant combinations of flavours in a wok.

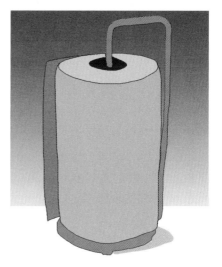

KITCHEN ROLL

If you fry, drain the food on a plate lined with kitchen paper when you take it out of the pan. This can go a long way to cutting down your fat consumption – you will be surprised at the amount left behind on the paper.

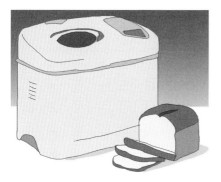

BREADMAKER

Although it's difficult to get your head around how one of these devices works, a breadmaker could be the best piece of kitchen equipment you'll ever buy. Preparing a loaf and putting it on to bake takes only a few minutes, your home will fill with

The healthiest shopping list in the world

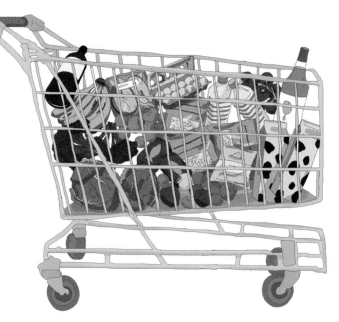

Bananas
Oranges
Grapefruit
Strawberries
Apples
Lemons
Kiwi fruit
Pineapple

Whole wheat flour
Whole wheat pasta
Brown rice
Whole grain cereals
Dried beans (soya, haricots, red kidney beans, lentils)

Sardines
Salmon steaks
Mackerel
Tuna steaks
Chicken breasts (skin removed)
Lean beef
Liver
Eggs

Olive oil
Sunflower oil
Whole black peppercorns
Vinegar (wine or balsamic)

Bottled water
Skimmed milk
Red wine
Green tea

Herbal infusions
Fruit tea

Nuts: walnuts, almonds, peanuts
Dried apricots
Sunflower seeds
Raisins
Olives
Jaffa cakes - they're a very good energy source!

Cabbage
Broccoli
Carrots
Green peppers
Spinach

Tomatoes
Aubergines
Red chilli peppers
Asparagus
Potatoes
Sweet potatoes
Onions

Olive oil spread
Low-fat cheese
Fat-free yoghurt

Root ginger
Parsley
Basil
Garlic

What not to eat

Although anybody's healthy eating plan will be complex and individually tailored to their needs, body type and metabolism, there are certain basic guidelines that apply to everybody. These concern what foods should be avoided.

REFINED SUGAR

This is the most common of 'empty calorie' foods, which are high in calorific value but deliver no nutritional value whatsoever. Sugar provides fuel but contributes enormously to weight gain as the body stays hungry for nutrients and will want more food long before the calories are burnt off. Try and cut down on sugary drinks (the average can of soft drink contains nine teaspoons of sugar), put less sugar in tea and coffee or switch to a sugar substitute, and avoid sugar-rich desserts and pastries.

SALT

Salt is dangerously on the rise in western diets. This isn't because of what you sprinkle on your plate or put in cooking, but because so many processed and snack foods contain far more sodium than they used to. Excess salt can lead to dangerously raised blood pressure and, eventually, congestive heart failure. Look for labels that advise 'low sodium' or 'salt-free'.

BUTTER AND FULL-FAT DAIRY PRODUCTS

These are loaded with saturated fats that dangerously raise your cholesterol levels. Butter is best avoided altogether – olive oil spread is a delicious and healthy alternative – and low or non-fat dairy products are good healthy substitutes.

TRANS FATS

These are found only in processed foods and will lurk behind the name 'partially hydrogenised oils'. Steer clear of anything with this on the label as trans fats do little other than drastically increase your cholesterol levels. Which is not good.

PROCESSED FOODS

Stay away from them in general, as the rise in the consumption of processed foods – especially among younger or single men – is one of the big factors in the rise of obesity rates. These foods deliver too many empty calories for not nearly enough nutritional value, encouraging people to overeat.

Fat, cholesterol and obesity and how they conspire to kill you

Being fat is no joke. In fact, it's so not funny that questions are being asked by Western governments about the size of their nation's waistlines.

During the last few years, our attitudes to weight gain have changed. People no longer talk about a fat child being a healthy child or believe that it's perfectly acceptable for the average man to put on a bit as he gets older. Even so, the rich West in general, especially men and children, are getting fatter. So much so that the UK government is considering passing legislation about food advertising and food standards.

This will no doubt do some good, but the real problem is that while the medical profession and a couple of government departments are aware of the growing (in more ways than one) dangers of obesity, the general public has yet to catch up. More and more men in the UK are getting bigger and bigger, and 'overweight' is spilling into 'obese' at a rate fast approaching epidemic proportions. These days 40 per cent of men

Fat or fit? Find out

The body mass index, or BMI, is how you work out whether the weight you're carrying around falls into the realm of healthy or health hazard. Based on calculations using your height and weight, it gives you an index number that can be measured against a set of international standards. It's a very simple formula:

1. Work out your weight in kilograms (kg) and your height in metres (m).

2. Square your height in metres (multiply it by itself).

3. Divide that figure into your weight.

4. The resulting number is your BMI.

If you weigh 90 kg and your height is 1.86 m, calculate your BMI thus:

1.86 x 1.86 = 3.4596; divide that figure into 90, which gives you a BMI of 26.0145.

What the figures mean is:

BMI of less than 18	Underweight
BMI between 18 and 25	Healthy
BMI between 25 and 30	Overweight
BMI of over 30	Obese

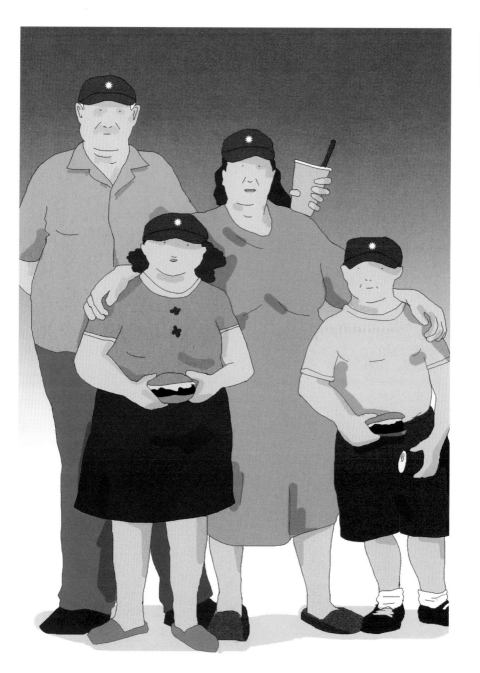

The Fatt family. Attractive, no? And to think that governments want to get rid of people like them.

Cholesterol explained

Cholesterol is vital to your body cells as it moves fats around the bloodstream to deliver them to the body's tissues.

It is produced by the liver, which also disposes of unwanted fat-carrying cholesterol that is delivered back to it.

Cholesterol in your body is of two different types: low density lipoprotein (LDL) and high density lipoprotein (HDL).

LDL is dangerous as it is of a low enough density to penetrate artery walls and leave fatty deposits, which in time can build up and cause blockage.

HDL, because it is of a much higher density, cannot get into the artery walls. It carries fat around the bloodstream and returns to the liver, bearing any unwanted fat for disposal. HDL actually works to keep your arteries clear.

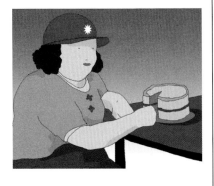

in the UK over the age of 30 are overweight and ten per cent of men over the age of 40 are officially obese. And these figures are growing and moving down the age scale. A man with a body mass index (see page 126) of over 25 is clinically overweight, if that figure rises to above 30 he is obese.

After smoking, excess weight is probably the biggest single cause of days lost for sickness in the UK, as it can lead to a number of different complaints. These go way beyond the heart disease and high blood pressure we discussed in detail earlier (see chapter 1), and diabetes (see pages 142–47) is only one of the potential dangers. Being overweight makes you more liable to cancer of the colon and it is also directly related to

the likelihood of gallstones – the bigger you are the bigger your chances. Obesity can interfere with your sleep, not just from the sheer awkwardness of a big belly but dangerously so. The risks of an alarming condition called sleep apnoea – in which the sleeper stops breathing for several seconds at a time – are much greater among the overweight. Sleep apnoea causes oxygen levels in the blood to drop and can put a severe strain on the heart. There will be serious stress on your joints and tendons, too, as a result of carrying extra weight. Your ankles and knees work hard enough as it is; making them support more weight can, over time, wear away the cartilage that cushions the joints. Increased load-bearing can also

Family history plays a big part in determining your cholesterol profile. If your father, his father and his father all suffered from heart disease, you will, too. So do something about it. It's not inevitable that you'll have a heart attack if you live properly and take expert advice. Find out about Statins. They could save your life.

Belly belly bad

When men put on weight any excess fat is more likely to collect on their bellies than anywhere else. This can be particularly bad news for more reasons than simply making you look like a slob. Belly fat is far more dangerous than fat on, say, your upper arms, as the chances of it turning your blood acid by releasing fatty acids into the liver is much higher. Abdominal fat is also far more efficient at releasing cholesterol into your bloodstream. It can be doubly dangerous if you're a diabetic, as belly fat produces a hormone that blocks the action of insulin, the hormone that regulates blood sugar levels. Tests have shown that men with a waistline of over 100 cm (40 in) are five times more likely to suffer heart disease than their slimmer contemporaries.

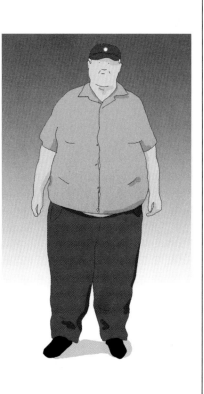

cause a swelling of the tendons, notably the Achilles tendon in the lower leg. And don't forget back pain. By the time they reach the age of 40 most men have suffered back pain at some point, and much of this could have been avoided if it weren't for the weight of the belly that the lower spine has to support.

High levels of dangerous cholesterol are linked to being overweight, too. Cholesterol is a fatty substance produced by the liver from fat taken in as food – particularly animal fat and dairy products – and is transported round the body in the bloodstream. A certain level of one type of cholesterol known as high density lipoprotein (HDL) is vital to the body for hormone production. However, another type of cholesterol, called low density lipoprotein (LDL), can accumulate in the arteries and eventually build up to narrow and block blood vessels. Being overweight means you are far more likely to have high cholesterol levels, due to the amount of fat you have in your system.

The average weight of British men has increased by nearly five per cent over the past decade. Older men, in particular, are among the overweight because although their calorie requirements drop with age, it's easy for their food intake to remain the same. Obesity is something that has to be taken seriously.

How much is safe?

All men over the age of 30 should get their cholesterol levels checked every three years, more often if they are overweight or have a history of heart problems.

The test should involve not just a reading of the overall level of cholesterol in your bloodstream, but should analyse the amounts of LDL and HDL.

Cholesterol is measured in milligrams (mg) of cholesterol in decilitres (dL) of blood. Ideally, your overall reading should be under 200 mg/dL; anything over 240 mg/dL and you are at serious risk of heart disease.

Your LDL reading should be under 100 mg/dL and your HDL reading should be over 40 mg/dL – the higher the latter figure, the less likely your risk of heart disease.

The ten easiest ways to lose weight

1 Drink more water

It'll fill you up but supply no calories at all.

2 Drink colder water

Your body will burn calories warming itself up after an internal dousing of icy water.

3 Eat more slowly

It takes the brain about 20 minutes to register that the stomach is full. Because we eat many meals much faster than this, we tend to go past the natural point of not needing any more.

4 Eat more often

Yes! Your digestive system can cope much better with several small meals a day – five is the ideal number – than it can with one or two large ones.

5 Eat a 'proper' breakfast

People who are overweight are much more likely to be skipping breakfast than those who are slim. This is because after not eating during the night the body needs fuel, so the temptation to snack until lunchtime is difficult to resist.

6 Eat less

It might seem obvious, but the trend in restaurants and fast-food joints to give bigger and bigger portions is causing us to overeat without realising it.

7 Chew longer

It's the chewing action that the brain associates with eating, so spending longer chewing each bite goes a long way to convincing the brain that you are full.

8 Stop if you feel full

Don't go past the point of being comfortable just to finish something or because you couldn't resist the sweet trolley.

9 Eat more fibre

It'll boost your metabolism to burn fat faster.

10 Read labels carefully

'Low fat' or 'fat free' can often mean a carb content that is packed with calories, and '90 per cent fat free' means that the other 10 per cent is fat.

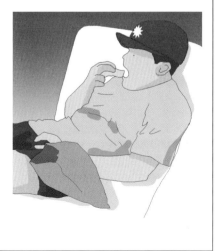

Why should you exercise?

Dieting may be the quickest route to better health, but regular exercise is the best way to maintain good health and to keep yourself fit.

It's easy to confuse being healthy and being fit, as it is perfectly possible to be one without being the other – there are plenty of fit fat people in the world, just as there are unfit health freaks. But to know the difference and to be both is to give yourself the best chance possible of a long, fulfilled and active life. Being fit goes a long way to guarding you against cardiovascular disease, makes you feel physically better to approach life with less strain, and helps to keep your mental processes sharp. Plus, of course, exercise keeps your weight down, so you'll not only feel better but look better, too.

Regular exercise gets more important for men as they get older, because to carry on living the life you are used to, you have to work at maintaining strength in muscles and tendons. In fact, when you are approaching

The calorie counter

All exercises or activities produce different levels of calorific burn, and it is important to choose the one most suitable for your desired fitness programme. The figures below are a guide to how much physical effort each activity requires. All numbers refer to calories burnt per hour of continuous activity.

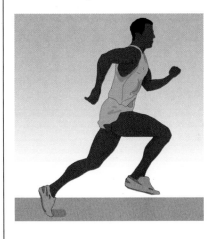

Squash	750
Swimming	350/750
Running (13 kph/8 mph plus)	700
Aerobics (medium to high intensity)	550
Cycling (16 kph/10 mph)	500
Circuit training	500
Jogging (11 kph/7 mph or less)	500
Basketball	450
Football	350
Badminton	350
Walking (briskly)	300
Yoga	300
Sex (enthusiastically)	200

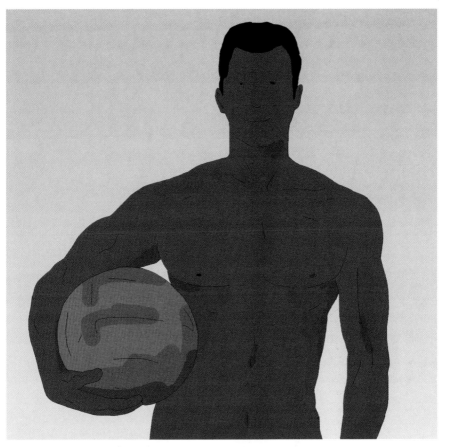

It's not called a medicine ball for nothing, you know. Exercise makes you fit, which helps you to maintain good health. Just don't try to swallow the ball, it's not that kind of medicine.

Any exercise is better than none. You may feel self-conscious in a gym and that's good, because it'll drive you on to get fit, faster. Nobody likes a lard ass.

old age, not exercising becomes something of a vicious circle – without working to stay fit you will rapidly lose strength, and the less strength you have the less you will be able to work at keeping fit.

Any exercise is better than none at all. If you've lived an almost totally sedentary life thus far, then look for things you can do that will increase your physical activity but won't be a danger to you at this stage. Walking instead of driving, taking the stairs instead of the lift, getting off the bus a couple of stops earlier and so on are ideal ways to begin to up your exercise quota – or, in some cases, to get started in the first place! If you are going to take on a workout programme or get into an activity such as jogging or cycling, the golden rule is to be sensible. If you have a history of heart problems or are diabetic, consult your doctor for advice on what is best for you. Otherwise, start out slowly to establish what your capabilities are and how much more you have to do to safely stretch your muscles.

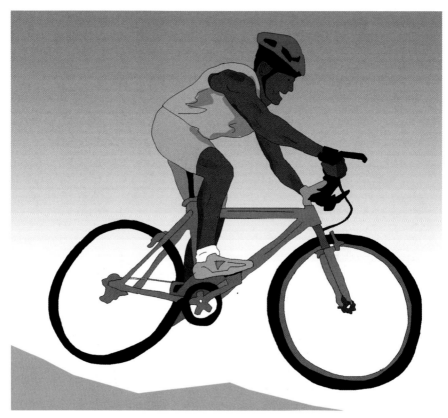

Cycling is a great aerobic exercise and you get to wear silly clothes, too! If you need any persuading about the benefits of cycling, see Lance Armstrong.

How exercise keeps your weight down

1
Working out beyond the energy you normally expend puts immediate strain on the muscles you are using

8
After a period of regular exercising you begin to noticeably lose weight

2
Those muscles require added fuel, in exactly the same way your car would if it was being driven faster

7
As the sequence continues – after about 20 minutes of exercising – your cardiovascular system starts to draw on the reserves of fat stored all over your body

3
Fat is the most obvious internal fuel and it has to be delivered to the muscles concerned

6
As you start to burn calories, increased energy levels allow you to exercise with increased intensity, requiring more fuel to the muscles and so perpetuating the cycle

4
As you exercise, your heart begins to beat faster to pump more blood round to make sure this energy supply reaches the muscles

5
You begin to breath deeper to supply the oxygen needed to metabolise this fat into energy

Warming up and cooling down

Nearly half of all amateur sporting injuries are caused by participants not warming up properly before they hurl themselves into the fray. The proportion rises sharply as said players get older and the body needs to be nursed into action with considerably more care and attention. The most common injuries suffered by the un-warmed-up are sprains, strains, muscle tears, bruised muscles and damaged joints. Almost as worrying is the fact that if you go onto the field of play without warming up your performance will be much less immediately effective than that of a player who has done some preparation. As regards keeping fit, if you warm up properly before you work out then you will immediately start burning fat, as opposed to 10 minutes into the exercise. The rules for warming up are simple:

1 Pulse warmers

These are short sets of intense activity – cycling, skipping, sprinting, spot running, jumping jacks – designed to increase your heart rate from its resting rhythm of approximately 70 beats per minute to nearer the 150 or so it will be when you start exercising for real. Pulse warmers reduce the risk of heart stress, loosen the muscles by decreasing their viscosity and allow increased oxygen to be delivered immediately, counteracting the breathlessness often experienced at the start of a workout.

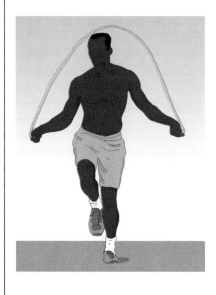

2 Stretching

This relaxes the fibres of the now-loosened muscles, and protects against strains and sprains. Stretching also cuts down the possibilities of minor bruising, as the looser the muscle tissue the greater its ability to absorb pressure or impact. You should perform three sets of stretches on each major muscle group, stretching slowly and comfortably and holding for 15 seconds. Never bounce into a stretch.

3 Mobility exercises

Also known as ballistic exercises, these loosen the joints by relaxing their connecting tendons and increasing the flow of natural lubrication. On-the-spot jumping is for knees and ankles, bending and rotation works for the hips and waist – stripper-style if you fancy it – and arms should be rotated at the shoulders and the elbows, while you waggle the hands at the wrists.

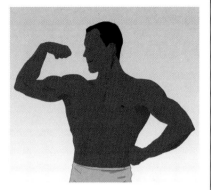

4 Skill rehearsal

When you see professionals like tennis players or cricketers or footballers miming playing shots or bowling or kicking before they start playing, they are rehearsing their skill. It's a mental warm-up that activates the muscle memory, so that by the time the contest begins the actions are subconscious rather than conscious.

COOLING DOWN

Just as important as warming up, cooling down brings the body back to normal after a period of intense physical activity. It is one of the most neglected aspects of amateur sporting performance or gym workouts. While not cooling down properly won't actually do you any lasting damage, you will feel a great deal better the next day if you take ten minutes to readjust. The reason for this is that while your muscles are working hard they produce lactic acid as their cells break down glucose for energy, and the acid goes on accumulating for a

brief while after the activity has stopped. Because you are no longer working out, the lactic acid does not get fully pumped away from your muscles and remains there to cause the soreness and stiffness often felt after exercise. Cooling down (or warming down, as it is also called) removes this lactic acid from your muscles. Again, the rules are simple:

1 Jog, jump, skip, cycle at a progressively decreasing pace, to bring your heartbeat gradually back to normal.

2 Gradually decrease energetic mobility to disperse lactic acid in muscles.

3 Stretch gently and you should feel your muscles begin to tighten as they return to their normal density.

4 Take a hot shower to complete the physical relaxation of your muscles and cool yourself down mentally.

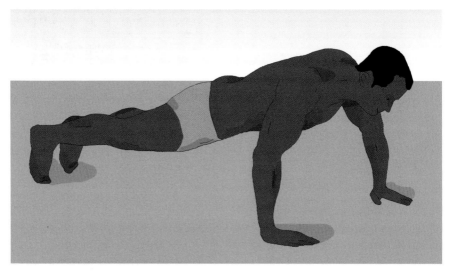

Once you've got fit, you can fall face-first to the floor and not hurt yourself! You can get bit parts in war movies because of your ability to 'drop and give me fifty, mister!'

The good workout guide

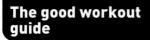 Set yourself realistic goals, both short term and long term.

Choose an activity or routine that you can a) keep up without becoming frustrated or disheartened; and b) fits in with your life so you don't keep finding excuses not to do it.

Avoid boredom by varying your routine – this also keeps your body working harder as you'll be using different muscles.

Eat a high carb snack an hour or so before you start exercising so you don't run out of energy during your workout.

Exercise with somebody – you can spur each other on and keep each other company.

Drink plenty of water before, during and after your workout.

Keep a record of what you are doing so that you can chart your progress.

Whatever you decide to do, exercising for increased fitness, muscle building or weight loss isn't quantum physics. For increased fitness or stamina – for instance, if you're training to run a marathon – you have to build up the time spent on the activity by gradually increasing your exertion, adding a quarter of an hour or so a week. If you want to build muscles, work those muscles to a point just beyond comfortable – you will know when that is – by adding greater weights. That way, over a surprisingly short space of time, the muscles get bigger to cope with what is expected of them. As regards weight loss, all you need to remember is that calories expended have to outnumber calories consumed, so pick an activity that satisfies this formula (see box, page 132) and make sure you don't start overeating to compensate.

One of the best ways to make sure you keep up with the exercise once you have started is to establish a routine; you will be able to work with much less perceived effort. Set aside a regular time, like first thing in the morning or lunchtime, and stick to it so that it becomes 'something you do'. People will come to respect that time as yours. Make sure you get the correct gear, paying particular attention to shoes. Sports shoe design is a science these days and styles are so sports-specific you could actually do yourself a great deal of harm by, for instance, running in tennis shoes or playing squash in basketball boots.

And finally, don't forget to warm up and cool down properly as described on pages 136–37.

RICE for injuries

The best basic way to treat sports injuries is with a simple formula known as RICE: rest, ice, compression, elevation. Of course, if your injury doesn't respond to this treatment you should seek professional advice.

1 Rest

Stop what you are doing as soon as something hurts and try not to use the injured area or put any weight on it for 24 hours.

2 Ice

Apply ice to bruises or sprains to bring down swelling and relieve pain. Ice cubes in a plastic bag wrapped in a towel make an effective ice pack.

3 Compression

Elastic or compression bandages applied to the injury give support and help to prevent swelling.

4 Elevation

Further control swelling by raising the affected area above your heart to reduce the likelihood of blood and fluid collecting there.

You need knees

Given the amount of poundage your knees have to bear, the amount of times they have to bear it – every time you take a step pretty much all your body weight is on your hinging knee – and the degree of balance they have to exert, the knee joint is a miracle of engineering. But it's precisely because of that they are the most vulnerable of all your joints. Some of the most common sports injuries involve the knees, and much of what is described below can be applied to the tendons and cartilage in other joints such as the ankles and elbows.

WHAT'S THE WORST THAT CAN HAPPEN?

Strain Overstretching the tendons in and around the joint will cause a strain, which is a relatively temporary condition and can be relieved by massage and gentle flexing

Sprain This will be caused by a sudden and unnatural twisting of the joint in which the ligaments are stretched. A period of RICE (see page 139) will usually cure any sprain.

Torn Ligament Considerably worse than a sprain, as the pressure has been so great on the ligament that it has ruptured. They come about as the result of a blow to the joint or severe twisting, and are often accompanied by an audible popping sound. Torn ligaments will either be repaired surgically or the limb will be immobilized by a cast while healing takes place naturally. It is the tearing of the cruciate ligaments in the knee that is an all too common injury among professional sportsmen, and will keep them out of action for up to a year.

Torn Cartilage Once again a common sports injury – particularly among basketball players – and caused by sudden twisting with the foot planted rigid. It is treated exactly the same as a torn ligament, with either surgery or enforced inactivity.

Runner's knee

Technically known as Chrondromalacia patellae, this is one of the most common ailments to affect long distance runners. This is a gradually occurring condition, in which the cartilage under the kneecap becomes inflamed impeding its mobility and causing friction against the already swollen cartilage.

SYMPTOMS

A stabbing pain under the kneecap. Noticeable when running, kneeling, going downstairs or sitting with knee bent for a long time.

CURE AND PREVENTION

Rest. Exercise quadriceps (front thigh muscle) and build up mileage slowly.

STOP!

Do not run if in pain.

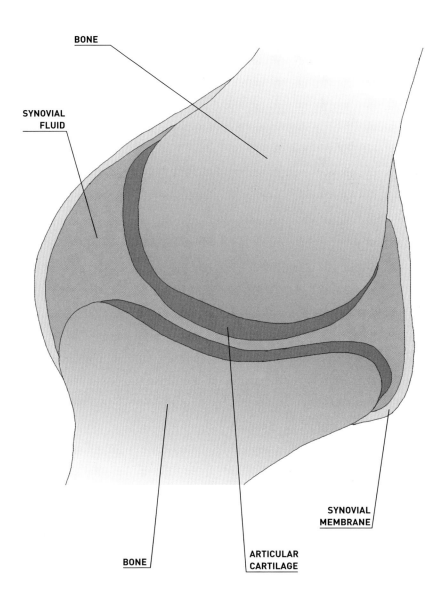

BONE

SYNOVIAL FLUID

SYNOVIAL MEMBRANE

BONE

ARTICULAR CARTILAGE

Diabetes: the sugar trap

Diabetes is an increasingly common condition among men and women in the UK, yet it is estimated that there are over a million diabetics who don't know they've got it simply because they don't understand the condition.

Diabetes mellitus, to give it its full name, is a condition in which either the pancreas fails to produce enough, or any, of the hormone insulin, or the body is resistant to the action of insulin. Insulin is vital to the functioning of the muscles; it is what allows your muscle cells to absorb the blood sugar (or glucose) created by your liver from starchy or sugary foods and to use it as energy to power movement. If the muscles aren't getting enough glucose, the body has to find other sources of energy, so it compensates by metabolising all the fat and protein it can locate – which is why diabetics can unexplainedly lose weight. The unused glucose can reach dangerously high levels in the bloodstream.

There are two types of diabetes: type 1 (insulin-dependent) diabetes and type 2 (non-insulin-dependent) diabetes –

Types of diabetes

TYPE 1 DIABETES

This occurs when, for currently unknown reasons, your pancreas just stops producing insulin. Although it is sometimes known as 'juvenile-onset diabetes', because it usually develops in childhood, it can strike anybody at any time. Type 1 is also referred to as 'insulin-dependent diabetes', because for the rest of your life you have to give yourself a daily insulin injection to regulate your blood sugar levels.

TYPE 2 DIABETES

Often called 'adult-onset diabetes', this type usually only hits people over the age of 35, although the age of diagnosis is getting lower all the time. Type 2 is also referred to as 'non-insulin dependent diabetes' because the pancreas produces insulin although the body cannot use it effectively. Although it can affect anybody, you are far more likely to suffer from type 2 diabetes if you are a) overweight; b) eat poorly, with a lot of refined sugar in your diet; or c) don't get enough exercise. Insulin injections may not be necessary if your blood sugar can be regulated by a change of diet or lifestyle.

You are at increased of diabetes if ...

You are over 35

Type 2 diabetes is most common in older people but the age range is falling and cases in twenty-somethings are becoming more frequent.

It runs in the family

Although diabetes isn't always passed down, the more diabetic relatives you have, and the closer they are to you on the family tree, the more likely you are to be affected.

You are overweight

Over three-quarters of all the men in the UK with type 2 diabetes are overweight.

You are of African-Caribbean or Indian origin

Nearly a quarter of all Indian men are diabetic, and if you are of African-Caribbean descent in the UK, you are between three and five times more likely to become diabetic than your Caucasian counterparts.

You don't exercise

Leading a sedentary lifestyle can vastly increase your chances of diabetes.

You have a lot of sugar in your diet

It messes with your blood glucose levels and eventually affects your insulin production capabilities.

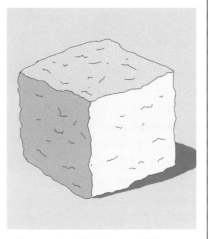

A sugar cube. Fine for horses, OK in moderation in beverages.

three-quarters of sufferers in the UK are type 2 diabetics. Type 1 is the most dangerous form of diabetes and occurs when the pancreas produces little or no insulin. The shutdown usually happens suddenly, for unknown reasons, and although it can occur at any time of life the great majority of cases are in people under the age of 40. There is no cure and the condition can be managed only by daily injections of insulin for life. Although alternative methods of treatment are under development in the USA – skin patches, capsules and inhalable insulin powder – as yet intravenous injection is the only way to take insulin.

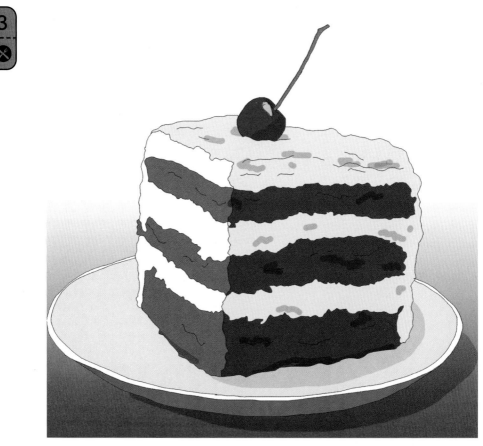

Hmmmmmmm. A cherry worth popping and then devouring the rest of the cake. Oh, but it's not really good for you, so share it with a friend. Or something.

Type 2 diabetes is far more common and, due to diet and lifestyle choices in the developed world, has been on the rise in recent years. It is often called adult-onset diabetes as it tends to strike late into adult life – 40-plus – but it is now regularly affecting people in their twenties or even younger. In type 2 diabetes the pancreas still produces insulin but the body is incapable of making use of it. This form of diabetes may not need insulin injections, although they cannot be ruled out completely, and as it is usually a result of being overweight and under-exercised type 2 can often be controlled with simple lifestyle changes.

Unhealthy eating of too much sugar and fat creates huge amounts of glucose that can overwhelm even a healthy system. The insulin present cannot make use of all this glucose, so it sloshes around in the

Diabetes facts

About three per cent of the population of the UK has been diagnosed as diabetic at any one time. It is believed that as many again may have the condition without being aware of it.

Diabetes is an equal-opportunity condition, affecting as many men as women worldwide.

Seventy-five per cent of those affected are type 2 diabetics.

The older you are the more likely you are to be diagnosed as diabetic.

Nearly ten per cent of the NHS's annual budget is devoted to diabetes and diabetes-related conditions.

Diabetes can lead to problems with your eyes, feet, kidneys, heart, stomach and lower limbs.

Diabetics are three times more likely to suffer heart disease than non-diabetics.

Diabetes affects nerve endings, particularly in the feet, and around five per cent of diabetics develop foot ulcers each year – it's the most common reason for diabetics to seek medical attention.

Nearly 25 per cent of diabetic men become impotent.

Diabetes causes more deaths in the UK than either breast cancer or AIDS.

Diabetics are entitled to free eye tests and free prescriptions.

Diabetics have to declare their condition when applying for motor insurance.

The average age at which diabetes is diagnosed is 51.

Diabetes affects the capillaries around the eyes – in the UK, more cases of blindness are attributed to diabetes than to any other single cause.

Diabetes can be controlled by diet and exercise and doesn't necessarily mean insulin injections for the rest of your life.

bloodstream turning dangerously toxic. Poor eating habits are also liable to lead to an accumulation of body fat, which has been directly linked to type 2 diabetes. Fat creates a rise in a hormone called resistin that works to prevent insulin getting glucose to the muscle cells. Changing bad eating habits, exercising and losing weight can contribute so much to the management of type 2 diabetes that the sufferer may not need to take on board extra insulin, although sometimes doctors prescribe medication that helps insulin work.

Although diabetes is not curable in the conventional sense, it is manageable. If you need insulin injections, they will so quickly become part of your daily routine you will virtually cease to notice them; and making changes to your lifestyle will benefit your entire state of health. Most type 2 diabetics can continue to enjoy a drink or the sweet trolley or a bar of chocolate, provided they are careful and balance it elsewhere.

The most common warning signs of diabetes are unquenchable thirst, tiredness (especially after a meal), sudden weight loss, frequent urination and blurred vision. If you think you might be diabetic, it is vitally important to get the condition diagnosed without delay. Untreated diabetes can cause all sorts of related problems such as nerve damage (the majority of lower limb amputations are diabetes-related, as are foot ulcers), sight problems (more cases of blindness in the UK are attributed to diabetes than anything else – diabetics are entitled to free eye tests) or kidney disease (a quarter of all diabetics suffer from kidney complaints). And the worrying thing as far as you're concerned is that undiagnosed diabetics are much more likely to be male than female, as men in general go to the doctors far less.

Diabetes is on the rise in the UK and the USA. Adult-onset diabetes used to affect people over the age of 35, but that median age is lowering, rapidly. That's because more and more people under that age are becoming overweight, with more cases of obesity being reported than at any time previously. If you're fat, you are going to be sick.

What you can do for yourself

If you have recently been diagnosed as diabetic, these are some of the things you can do to make your new lifestyle easier:

Do not be embarrassed by your condition.

Give up smoking.

Take a regular amount of exercise – how much depends on the individual.

Avoid eating sweet foods, unrefined carbohydrates (starch) and saturated fat.

Eat more fibre.

Get into a routine of regularly monitoring your blood sugar levels.

Strike up a good relationship with your doctor – you will be seeing a lot more of him or her

If you are type 1, make sure you establish an unbreakable routine for injecting your insulin.

Always carry identification that clearly describes your condition.

Educate those around you at home and at work to recognise hypoglycaemia (dangerously low blood sugar) and hyperglycaemia (dangerously high blood sugar), and to know what to do if either occurs.

If you play organised sports, make sure your teammates and the controlling bodies are aware of your condition; a few sports do not allow diabetics to compete.

SOME USEFUL CONTACTS

DIABETES UK
10 Parkway
London NW1 7AA
www.diabetes.org.uk
0845 1220 2960

DIABETES SPORTS & EXERCISE ASSOCIATION
www.diabetes-exercise.org

AMERICAN DIABETES ASSOCIATION
www.diabetes.org

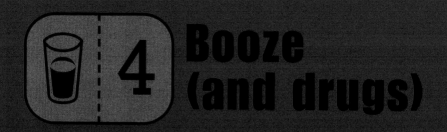

4 Booze (and drugs)

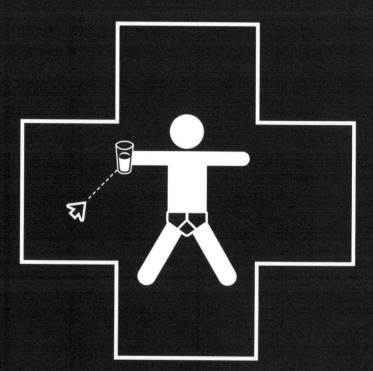

MOST OF US ENJOY A DRINK AND IT DOESN'T USUALLY DO US ANY HARM. BUT, IF IT GETS OUT OF CONTROL, ALCOHOL CAN DESTROY YOUR LIFE. DO YOU KNOW THE DIFFERENCE BETWEEN MODERATE AND EXCESSIVE DRINKING?

Enjoy a drink, do you?

Alcohol in moderation is unlikely to do you much harm. Indeed, it might even be beneficial. But to make it work for you, you have to fully understand it.

Most men like a drink on a pretty regular basis. In Western society, alcohol is the lubricant that oils the wheels of a vast number of social situations, helping people to unwind, open up and feel comfortable. A far-from-overindulgent one or two glasses of red wine a day has been shown to aid the circulation, cutting down the likelihood of heart disease or high blood pressure. Alcohol can also stimulate production of gastric juice and increase the appetite for food – hence wine really will make a meal taste better.

Alcohol's main effect on a man's body – the reason we all drink it – is that it relaxes us. Once alcohol has got into the brain via the bloodstream it suppresses certain natural impulses by interfering with the operation of the brain's neurotransmitters, the chemical messengers that trigger nerve impulses. As we drink, alcohol progressively affects different parts of the brain. Its immediate effect is to stifle the brain areas that inhibit our behaviour, enabling us to lighten up and stop feeling so anxious about practically everything. It's a pretty good feeling and taps into the pleasure controls of the lower midbrain, which are programmed to order us to repeat or prolong the experience. That is what makes it so difficult to 'just have the one'.

As you go on drinking, the levels of alcohol build up in your blood to have an increasing effect on your brain. (How much booze you've got sloshing around in your system is determined by milligrams of alcohol per 100 millilitres of blood. The maximum legal level for driving is 80mg alcohol/100ml blood.)

Once your inhibitions have gone, your coordination won't be far behind, and this

**Given alcohol's inhibition-lowering abilities, it isn't too surprising that in 25 per cent of unwanted pregnancies the women had drunk too much alcohol at the time of conception.
However, this figure is remarkable in a way, seeing what booze can do to a man's motor skills, erectile capabilities and sperm count.**

will manifest itself in slurred speech as well as a noticeable lack of motor skills – noticeable to most people other than yourself, that is. After drinking for an hour or so your blood/alcohol levels will be very high and you will feel flushed with euphoria and self-confidence as your pleasure centres go into overdrive. You couldn't possibly be talking too loudly and mostly incomprehensibly, or knocking things over. You've reached this point because it takes about an hour for your body to respond to the toxins you're assaulting it with and process them for excretion. This is why when you start drinking you go ages before urinating, then once you've started you seem to go every ten minutes as your body's self-preservation instincts keep the expulsion cycle going – you wouldn't visit the gents nearly so often if you were drinking pints of water. You will probably start to feel hungry after a couple of hours and four or five beers, as stimulation of the gastric juices kicks in.

Unfortunately, it's downhill from here. The more you drink now the more your brain starts to shut down, leading to progressive failure of the motor reflexes. You eventually reach a point at which you can't talk, you can't walk and your coordination is so shot you can't look at things without them

The booze line

The following scenario illustrates how alcohol affects the casual drinker over the course of an evening in the bar. We have chosen a casual drinker as his tolerance level will be far nearer the national average than the heavy or regular drinker, who needs considerably more to advance along this course. We have chosen beer because it represents what most (male) social drinkers prefer, but each pint of it represents two units of alcohol, the same as a double measure of spirits or two glasses of wine.

THE FIRST BEER
You may immediately feel a small alcohol charge from this, but to no lasting effect. This is because only a small amount of alcohol goes straight into your bloodstream from your stomach, while most of it passes into the small intestine. If this was all you were drinking it would leave you with about 25mg alcohol/100ml blood.

THE SECOND BEER
It takes roughly an hour for the body to metabolise the alcohol in one pint of beer. Assuming, at this stage, you're drinking about one beer every 20 minutes, the levels soon build up as the alcohol passes into your bloodstream without being 'cleaned' out. After the second beer you will be up to about 75mg/100ml, and probably talking too much and too loudly as the alcohol decreases brain activity and represses your natural inhibitions.

The unit definition

A unit of alcohol is the equivalent of half a pint of regular strength beer or lager, a single measure of a spirit or a glass of wine. The recommended maximum is 21 units per week for men or 14 units per week for women. Anything over 50 or 35 units per week, respectively, is considered dangerous.

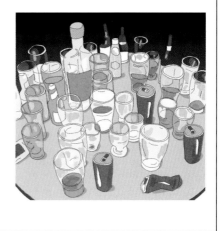

4

THE THIRD BEER

Alcohol levels will be up to 120mg/100ml after this – over the legal drink-drive limit of 80mg/100ml – as your body won't have processed any yet but it's still coming in. Your confidence levels are sky high by now as your brain has stopped responding to tension, anxiety and fear. With this comes slightly reduced self-control as your co-ordination starts to suffer – ironically, even if you notice this, it won't worry you because of the effects of the alcohol.

THE FOURTH BEER

You'll start going to the toilet as the body starts to expel the toxins you've been feeding it for the last hour and a half. With a blood alcohol level of around 140mg/100ml your co-ordination is really starting to suffer and your speech is affected. You'll be one of the last people to realise this, because by now you'll be labouring under the delusion that you are functioning more efficiently than usual.

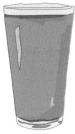
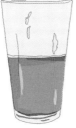

THE FIFTH BEER

You'll now be over 200mg/100ml, more than twice the legal limit, and you could be staggering slightly and starting to lose control of your emotions – extremes of affection or aggression are not uncommon. With your increasing lack of inhibition comes an enthusiasm to tell the truth, whether it is called for or not. You are feeling hungry because you have taken on virtually no nutrients at all during the last couple of hours, yet the frequency with which you are going to the toilet is depleting your system.

appearing to move. In short, you just want to curl up and close your eyes as your brain gives up the struggle to work things out. At some time before this happens you may even get the blues or be subjected to radical mood swings – remember, alcohol is a depressant and, ultimately, it will make you depressed.

When you wake up the next day, you won't feel too rested because this sort of sleep isn't really sleep at all, it's simply unconsciousness. The hangover you're probably suffering from is a combination of tiredness, dehydration from all that going to the loo to get rid of the toxins, and mild poisoning from the left-over toxins that your liver has yet to process. Drinking water before you go to bed helps with the dehydration, but it will only be a matter of time before the poisons clear. Incidentally, the fitter you are and the more efficient your cardiovascular system, the faster your recovery will be.

The booze line (cont.)

THE SIXTH BEER
You won't be making a lot of sense or any sudden movement by this point; 240mg/100ml leads to a noticeable slowing down of thought, word and deed.

THE SEVENTH BEER
Extreme confusion, disorientation and drowsiness set in, as your levels are up to 280mg/100ml. You will be having difficulty keeping the drink down as your system starts to rebel actively against the treatment you've subjected it to.

THE EIGHTH BEER
This could be the pint of no return. Your levels are over 300mg/100ml, more than four times the legal limit for driving. If you haven't thrown up yet, the effect on the nervous system and the brain will be so great it will pretty much shut down all but the vital functions. This will probably lead to passing out and maybe even an alcoholic coma. So much alcohol has entered the blood it will mean a case of alcohol poisoning that could take a few days to clear up.

Got a problem?

An awful lot of drinking goes on in the West, and most of the time it doesn't cause anybody any problems. Trouble is, for a significant number of people it does.

There isn't really any such thing as a safe level of drinking, not because all drinking is bad but simply because everyone has different danger levels. What doesn't change, though, are the signs and symptoms that somebody's drinking has turned from being a pleasure into being a pain. It can be a worryingly thin line between the two.

Before the physical conditions that can result from prolonged alcohol abuse (see following pages) take hold, heavy drinking can bring with it a raft of behavioural and psychological problems. No matter how we choose to acceptably use alcohol in social situations, it should never be forgotten that it is a powerfully addictive drug and it deserves to be treated with a bit more than casual respect.

As mentioned earlier, alcohol's stimulation of the brain's pleasure centres triggers the desire to repeat the experience. Coupled with the short-term discomfort of a hangover or coming down from an alcohol high, this makes it very easy to have another drink the morning after. A hair of the dog ... a bit of a livener ... we've all done it, but alleviating the after-effects can rapidly become a habit, and from there it's no distance at all between wanting a drink and needing a drink. Because the body's tolerance levels to alcohol rise over a fairly short space of time, it's easy for the amount you drink to go up quite quickly as well. That is how the escalating cycle of addiction kicks

Drinking statistics

Forty-five per cent of all crimes of violence involve alcohol.

The NHS spends £180 million a year on alcohol-related problems.

Twenty per cent of men admit to drinking too much.

One in three men drinks over the recommended maximum of 21 units a week.

One in six men admits to binge drinking – more than 12 units of alcohol in one session.

Men are nearly five times more likely to become alcohol-dependent than women.

One in four car accidents requiring ambulance attendance involves alcohol.

in, when you start drinking to make life bearable instead of making it better. The not-so-early warning signs of reaching this stage are cravings for alcohol, depression and discomfort about going through a day without a drink, or drinking first thing in the morning.

At this point, problems can occur that can affect your whole life. As your perceived tolerance for alcohol rises, it becomes very easy to get drunker than you are aware of in wholly inappropriate situations – at work, for

While alcohol is doing terrible things to your insides – particularly your kidneys and liver – it is making you look stupid, too. You might think that you're witty when under the influence of alcohol, but you're not. You're dumb. Believe it.

instance. Then, because you don't realise that your coordination and speech aren't what they ought to be, it won't be surprising if you get things wrong while labouring under the misapprehension that you are functioning perfectly well. You'll probably get argumentative and unreasonable, too, defending your mistakes with complete abandonment of logic.

Understandably, such behaviour isn't good for your employment prospects, personal relationships and dealings with the forces of law and order. In short, the world in general (excluding those who also view it through the bottom of a glass) will find you a bit of a pain in the rear and probably duck into a shop doorway when they see you coming. Which will really give you something to be pissed off about ... and now you've got a proper reason to have a drink.

Of course this a worst-case scenario, and it's unlikely to happen to the vast majority of drinkers. But the point of describing it here is that it could happen to practically any one of us, such is the power afforded to alcohol within modern society.

The four Ls

Alcohol dependency ultimately ends in the four Ls:

Liver
Your liver will bear the brunt of your drinking, until it packs up.

Lover
Your relationship will suffer as the result of your drinking.

Livelihood
If you can keep a job it won't be one that pays very well.

Law
As a persistent heavy drinker you are bound to end up on the wrong side of the law – probably sooner rather than later.

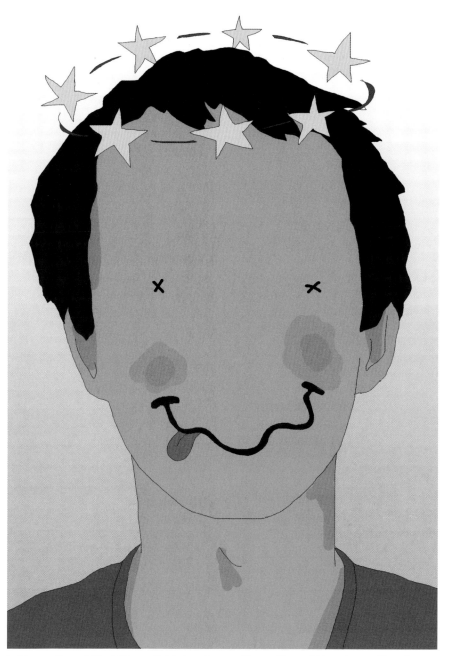

Is this you after a night out? Do you find that you have problems getting a girl to go home with you?

Quiz: have you got a drink problem?

Find out how you did on page 161.

1 In an average week do you drink:
a never;
b once or twice;
c most evenings;
d every evening and a few lunchtimes, too.

2 If you find you have no drink in the house do you:
a shrug and put the kettle on;
b swear and put the kettle on;
c go down to the off licence;
d go down to the bar.

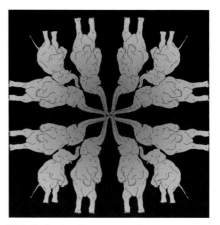

Pink elephants – if you can see them, you are drinking far too much.

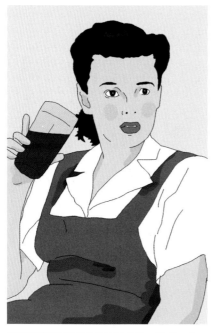

Judy Garland. Maybe she drank in order to get somewhere over the rainbow?

3 Do people you know – work colleagues, family, friends – comment on your drinking:
a never;
b occasionally;
c the morning after functions;
d frequently.

4 You are at a very good party/function do you stay until:
a the time you agreed to leave;
b the last train;
c the conversation runs out;
d the bar runs out.

5 You are at a function with a well-stocked bar, but also in attendance are people you ought to be impressing – the future in-laws, your kids' headteacher, the boss – do you:
a stick to soft drinks;
b drink in moderation;
c set out to do b) but end up somehow doing d);
d get legless.

6 Do you drink wine with a meal:
a never;
b on special occasions;
c only when out at dinner;
d whenever it is available.

7 If you've had a particularly stressful day do you:
a go for a run;
b have a glass of wine and talk it through with your partner;
c go down to the bar with your best mate;
d polish off a bottle of vodka by yourself.

8 If, at a party, the bar has got down to some very suspect-looking liqueur and 'wife beater' strength, horrible-tasting lager do you:
a not really notice because they've still got plenty of Evian;
b opt for a soft drink;
c go home;
d mix the two together and wonder why nobody else wants to sample your new cocktail.

9 You've woken up next to somebody you don't recognise how often:
a several times, but all of them were on transatlantic flights;
b not since university;
c not since you were last on holiday;
d sometimes you don't recognise the wife.

10 How would you describe your relationship with drink:
a non-existent;
b a mild flirtation;
c like having a mistress;
d lurrrrrve.

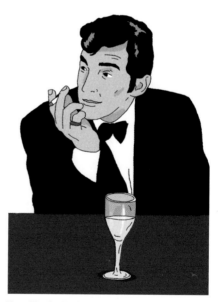

Dean Martin. No, it wasn't water in that glass. No, you can't sing 'That's Amore' very loudly.

4

'I put away so much I actually drank myself sober' and other drink-related nonsense

In spite of what professional footballers who put bin bags under their training tops tell you, you cannot sober yourself up by sweating out alcohol with physical exercise.

You may not be sleeping it off. The length of time alcohol stays in the average man's system is routinely underestimated and it is possible to get up the next day still well over the legal drink-drive limit.

Although a quick nip on a frosty day makes you feel warm inside, all it's doing is opening the blood vessels near the skin's surface and not increasing your true body tempera-ture. This false feeling of inner warmth can actually make you more vulnerable to seriously cold conditions.

Black coffee does not sober you up, it simply turns a sleepy drunk into a wide-awake drunk who is far more dangerous to himself and those around him.

Nobody drives 'better' when they've had a few.

Vodka does give you a hangover. The main cause of that dreadful feeling the next morning is dehydration, which all alcohol causes; the only possible advantage of vodka is it contains virtually no congeners, mildly toxic chemicals that are most prevalent in grape-related drinks (particularly red wine and brandy).

Women cannot out-drink men. The enzyme that breaks alcohol down before it can get into the bloodstream is four times more prevalent in men than in women, so women get drunk much quicker and more easily than we do.

A nightcap might help you get to sleep, but is very likely to wake you up in two or three hours when the alcohol has been metabolised by your liver and the resultant sugar rush breaks your sleep pattern.

It's impossible to have 'just a quick one after work'.

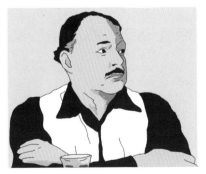

Ernest Hemingway. He wrote some good books. He drank a lot. He killed himself.

Dean Martin once quipped that, 'I drink because I have to. I'm not a drunk, my body is.' He was right. But he was also very cool. You, however, are not Dean Martin. So stop drinking so much.

What booze can do to you

Prolonged heavy drinking can do so much more than simply destroy your relationships, cost you your job, increase your weight and give you a permanently red face. Alcohol abuse is linked with a number of serious medical conditions.

LIVER DISEASE

Alcohol is broken down in the liver, but too much of it prohibits the organ's other functions. Fat builds up, which can lead to fibrosis (scarring of the liver), then alcoholic hepatitis and cirrhosis (see page 98), which can stop the liver working completely.

INFERTILITY

Drinking can adversely affect the sperm-producing cells within the testicles and inhibit the body's production of testosterone. Stopping drinking can usually reverse these conditions.

IMPOTENCE

Brewer's droop is a reality. Because alcohol affects the central nervous system it slows and dampens natural responses, one of which will be your erection.

HEART DISEASE

Prolonged heavy drinking carries greatly increased risks of high blood pressure, strokes or heart attacks.

PEPTIC ULCERS

The toxins in alcohol can cause severe irritation of the stomach and intestinal linings, which may result in ulcers.

CANCERS

The incidences of cancer of the mouth, larynx and throat are greatly increased in heavy drinkers.

Giving up gracefully

Unless you've got such an advanced alcohol problem that you need to put this book down and get off to your nearest AA meeting, cutting down drink from dangerous or anti-social levels to something less harmful isn't really that difficult. The problem most men have with cutting back on drinking is actually one of perception: they believe they will, a) put an end to their social life; b) look like a pussy; or c) not be able to function in social situations. None of these need to apply, and if you follow the simple guidelines given here it's relatively easy to rein in your drinking and avoid losing your footing on that slippery slope to serious problems.

Meet your friends for a drink an hour later than usual. It won't cut too much out of your socialising, but it could knock two or three drinks off your total for a session, which, over the course of a few weeks, could really add up.

Don't stand at the bar. You'll drink a great deal less if you have to fight your way up there every time you need a refill, plus it will remove the 'Same again?' pressure from the bar staff before you've even finished the last one.

Tail off towards the end of the evening by switching to non-alcoholic drinks. This one is tricky as you may

well be half cut, so approach it as if you are the designated driver.

Volunteer to be the designated driver. You'll drink much less and you get to go home when you want to.

Avoid drinking when you don't really have to, like at lunchtime or at halftime at the game. These single drinks may seem like nothing but they can start to add up.

Tell your friends you are cutting down. If they don't want to help you, or even stand in your way by taking the piss, then it might be time to get some new friends.

Make sure you have at least two days a week on the wagon. It'll prove to yourself you don't need to drink.

Get a hobby, something that doesn't involve meeting in a bar or going drinking afterwards. Carpentry is probably much more suitable than darts.

Don't keep strong liquor at home. If you're trying to cut down there's no point in getting it in. At least switch your home choice to low-alcohol beer or wine.

Change to longer drinks. Order those that take longer to finish, but aren't correspondingly higher in alcohol, like so many cocktails.

Alternate your drinks. Switch to a soft drink every two or three rounds during an evening. Changing to water reduces your risk of dehydration and a hangover.

Avoid people you only meet to drink with. If your only common interest with certain people is going to the bar, then it's probably best to avoid them for a while.

WHO YOU GONNA CALL?

ALCOHOLICS ANONYMOUS
PO Box 1, Stonebow House
North Yorkshire YO1 7NJ
24-hour helpline (0345) 697555

ALCOHOL ANONYMOUS (INT)
www.alcoholics-anonymous.org

AL-ANON
61 Great Dover Street
London SE1 4YF
(020) 7403 0888
www.hexnet.co.uk/alanon

ONLINE AA RECOVERY RESOURCE
www.recovery.org/aa

How did you score?

ALL As
You probably only did this quiz in order to show off how clean-living you are.

MOSTLY As
It's unlikely you will ever have a problem with alcohol as you don't seem to need it and are able to control your approach to it with admirable discipline.

MOSTLY Bs
If your Bs are mixed with As then you, too, have very little to worry about as you are the perfect social drinker. If they're mixed with Cs, though (especially on questions 3, 5 and 7) you should keep an eye on yourself.

MOSTLY Cs
You could have a problem, or the makings of one. You don't seem to be able to control your drinking too well and you may be kidding yourself that everything is OK – denial is a common attribute of people that drink at this level.

MOSTLY Ds
You are in serious trouble. Your drinking seems to be out of control, it is starting to impact on every aspect of your life and is doubtless affecting your health by now. You need to seek help a.s.a.p.

Drug related

Even the dimmest smackhead knows that illegal drugs don't do you a lot of good. What remains to be discussed, though, is how much bad they can do you.

Essentially, drugs mess you up, both in the long term and in the longer-than-immediate short term. They can creep up on you under socially acceptable circumstances without you knowing what's happening. Dependence on any illegal drug is much like it is for smoking or drinking. People repeatedly get high to avoid the comedown effects; or they convince themselves that they will function better under certain circumstances if they have a quick toot or a smoke, or believe that they can't function at all without it.

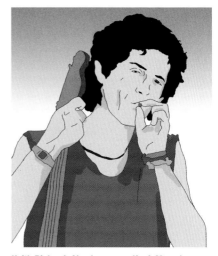

Keith Richard. Also known as Keef. Many have tried and all have failed to match his intake.

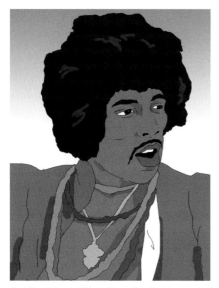

Jimi Hendrix could burn his guitar, but he couldn't handle his smack. Choked on his vomit.

The buying, selling and possession of illegal drugs immediately puts you on the wrong side of the law in the way going into a bar can't, and that can lead to devastating consequences. Furthermore, because illegal drugs are prepared under totally unregulated circumstances, unless it's something you grew yourself, it is virtually impossible for you know exactly what you are taking and what it has been mixed with. It's no coincidence that there is high level of pneumonia among heavy cocaine users as whatever the drug has been adulterated with – talcum powder, powdered milk, chalk dust and so on – will end up in the lungs. Another major health factor, again prevalent with cocaine use, is that the conditions under which drugs are taken can easily lead to infections: toilets, alley-ways and so on are hardly the most sanitary of situations.

It's often argued in defence of using drugs such as, say, marijuana and cocaine, that tobacco and alcohol, which remain legal, have far greater addictive properties and can do a staggering amount of damage to the human body. This is true, but it should be used as an argument against the latter rather than in favour of the former. And, if nothing else, fags and booze are difficult to overdose on, take a great deal of time to kill you and won't get you arrested for possessing them.

The drug debate is one that will run and run, but the best thing you can do for your health is to know exactly what is the worst that can happen.

MARIJUANA

After alcohol, this is the most popular recreational drug in the Western world. It is estimated that 60% of the people in the UK aged between 30 and 50 have tried marijuana at some point, a figure that goes up to 80% for those aged between 15 and 30. Marijuana is the dried leaves of the hemp plant and works as a mild sedative, producing a dreamy state of relaxation, heightening perception to, say, music or paintings and making the smoker liable to giggle at anything or nothing in particular; the passage of time loses significance. Side effects are a lack of coordination, hunger pangs and an inability to judge distances accurately (don't even think about driving). Prolonged usage can be a powerful demotivator. If marijuana is mixed with tobacco, the harmful effects of nicotine are added on to the effects of the drug. Because of lack of evidence that marijuana does any serious or lasting harm to the user and does

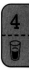

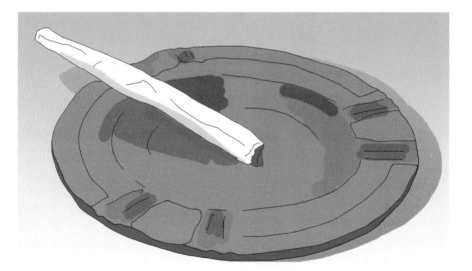

Just one joint. Never enough, but don't worry, it's not addictive. Neither does it automatically lead to any addiction to other, stronger drugs. Isn't the sky a bright blue? Where was I ...?

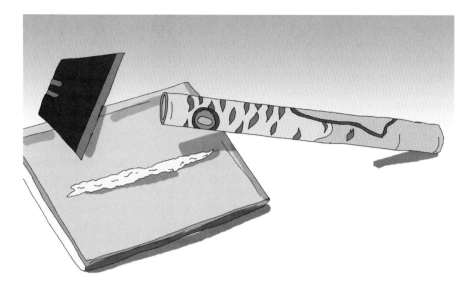

4

Cocaine. It used to be a rich man's drug, now anyone with the idea that they're fantastic can afford it. Why is it that people who take drugs use the ones that accentuate their character flaws?

not cause dangerous addiction, at the time of writing possession of a small amount for personal use had been decriminalised. This is widely believed to be the first step towards complete legalisation.

COCAINE

Originating from the leaves of the South American coca plant, cocaine has a numbing effect on the nerves close to the skin, and for that reason was once widely used as a local anaesthetic, particularly by dentists. When snorted, injected or smoked to get it into the bloodstream, the drug produces a rush of energy and an intense feeling of well-being. Cocaine abuse raises risks of a heart attack or stroke, as it constricts the arteries, raises blood pressure and causes an irregular heartbeat; sweating, nausea and a shortness of breath may go with this.

If snorted, it numbs the tissues inside the nose and prolonged abuse can destroy the septum (the wall in between the nostrils). Mostly, though, the effects of cocaine are psychological: aggressive or edgy behaviour is a side effect of the high, and regular usage can lead to paranoia. The rush of the high is followed by an equally dramatic comedown an hour or so later and can result in cravings to get high again. Prolonged cocaine use often causes insomnia, lack of focus, anxiety and depression.

CRACK COCAINE

Crack is cocaine purified into small pellets called rocks. With this form of the drug comes an intensification of everything that goes with regular cocaine. The rush of the high hits harder, lasts much less time – ten minutes or so – and the crash of the comedown is greater, as are the cravings for another hit. Long-term usage of crack cocaine can lead to severe psychological effects, including suicidal depression.

AMPHETAMINES

Speed, uppers, sulphate, whiz ... originating as appetite suppressants or slimming pills that were available perfectly legally, amphetamines are now almost totally illegal from manufacture to marketing. Very little of this clandestinely traded speed actually contains more than ten per cent amphetamine, the balance being practically anything that will bulk it up. These drugs act as stimulants by speeding up the cardiovascular system and will keep a tired man awake or boost normal energy levels. They can also bring on a rush of euphoria and a feeling of well-being. The comedown from speeding can cause depression and irritability, while prolonged use can lead to fatigue through lack of sleep and malnutrition due to a suppressed appetite.

HEROIN

A product of the opium poppy, heroin is one of the most speedily self-destructive drugs in popular usage. It is physically and psychologically addictive – state of dreamy

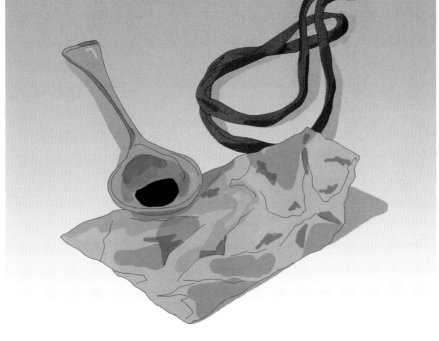

Heroin. Smack. Horse. Whatever you call it, this crap kills and isn't worth it. Dealers cut it with the kind of stuff that you clean toilets with and then you ingest it. What is wrong with you people?

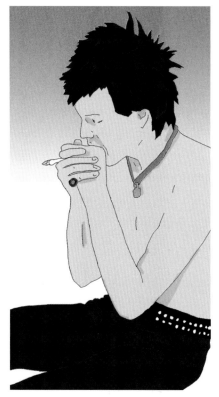

Sid Vicious. Too dumb to live. Became a junkie, killed his girlfriend and then himself.

ECSTASY

The current club drug of choice, MDMA (methylenedioxymethamphetamine), or ecstasy, is an amphetamine similar to speed, but supposedly without the raw edges that can easily turn speed users to violence. Ecstasy provides energy and euphoria and makes the user affectionate, dreamy and touchy-feely – not for nothing is it called the 'love drug'. While the long-term effects of regular usage are still being investigated – the drug hasn't been around long enough for anyone to know – in the short term, ecstasy interferes with the body's thermostat, raising the internal temperature and causing severe dehydration. The immediate results of frequent use are the same as caused by other amphetamines – not enough sleep and not enough to eat. Ecstasy has been linked with kidney and liver failure and brain damage, and there have been ecstasy-related deaths, but as such cases appear at random it has so far been impossible to draw conclusions or even to tell if the drug itself or what it had been adulterated with was responsible.

euphoria it produces and the harsh comedown afterwards both being powerful incentives to take another hit. Trouble is, the body quickly builds up a tolerance and requires larger and larger amounts. Obtaining heroin soon becomes all an addict's life is about. Heroin is normally injected, but as well as all the risks that involves – hepatitis, HIV and inflamed veins – long-term users are also liable to kidney disease and liver disorders.

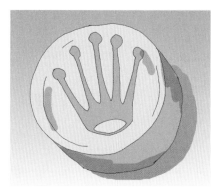

Ecstasy. It makes you love people too dumb to dance who wave their arms around instead.

LSD

Acid, or, to give it its chemical name, lysergic acid diethylamide, is a strong mind-altering, chemically manufactured substance that affects the user's perceptions of sound, colours, spatial relationships, shapes, time and movement to provide a genuinely alternative way of looking at the environment. If all goes well, an acid trip can be something of an incredible journey. However, if it is a 'bad trip', and there's no way of telling which it will be, it can be a truly terrifying experience. The long-term results of acid over-indulgence are considerably more scary than that: because LSD was designed as a psychiatric drug, it affects the brain and over time can lead to paranoia, depression and schizophrenia.

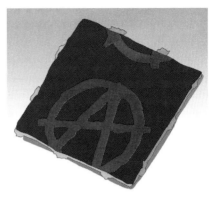

LSD was once considered to offer a path into a deeper consciousness. Now it's rat poison.

Who you gonna call?

DRUGAID
I Neville Street
Cardiff
CF1 8LP
(0800) 220794 or (01222) 383313

NARCOTICS ANONYMOUS
www.na.org

NICD
National Institute on Chemical Dependency
www.ni-cor.com

Illegal drug use is on the rise in every country that can afford it, and many that can't. And who benefits? Have you ever met a drug dealer that you liked? Do you really want to encourage that kind of ridiculous dressing up they do? So stop buying the stuff and get high on something else. Grow your own! Better still, grow up!

Natural remedies

Although there isn't a herbal cure to get you off drug or alcohol or nicotine dependency, there are a number of remedies you can take that will certainly help ease you through.

FOR STOPPING SMOKING

Kola nut Energises you and helps lift withdrawal-induced anxiety.

Ginger Cleans out your bloodstream.

Ginkgo Boosts your circulation.

Cubeb berry Rebuilds damaged lung tissue.

Saw palmetto berry Rebuilds physical and mental stamina.

Oat Combats post-smoking cravings and withdrawal pangs.

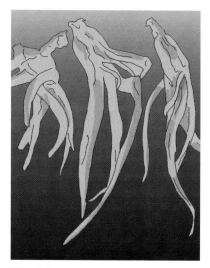

Natural ginseng. Very good for you and considered an aphrodisiac, too.

FOR STOPPING DRINKING

Milk thistle seed, turmeric or dandelion root Rejuvenate the liver.

Folic acid and thiamine Combat nutritional deficiencies brought on by drinking.

Evening primrose oil Compensates for alcohol's interference with the body's production of the essential fatty acid gamma linolenic acid.

Valerian root A tonic for the nervous system.

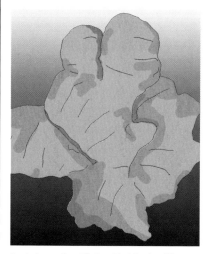

Root ginger. Great in tea, Thai food and beer.

FOR GIVING UP COCAINE, AMPHETAMINES OR ECSTASY

Kola nut Gives energy and calms the nervous system to reduce feelings of anxiety or paranoia.

Ginseng Combats fatigue.

Fo-ti root or eleuthero Builds stamina.

Milk thistle seed, turmeric or dandelion root Rejuvenate the liver.

FOR COMING OFF BARBITURATES OR DOWNERS

Magnesium Keeps you calm.

Milk thistle seed, turmeric or dandelion root Rejuvenate the liver

Garlic Cleanses the blood.

NB

If you are taking prescription drugs for your recovery, speak to your doctor before embarking on any course of natural remedies.

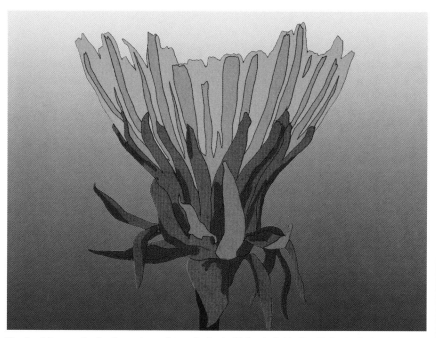

The dandelion can be drunk as a tea, eaten and mixed with burdock (don't ask). It also looks nice. It's not actually red, but we can't afford any other colours, remember?

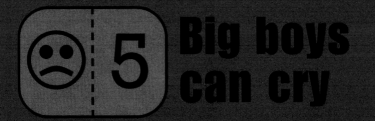

Big boys can cry

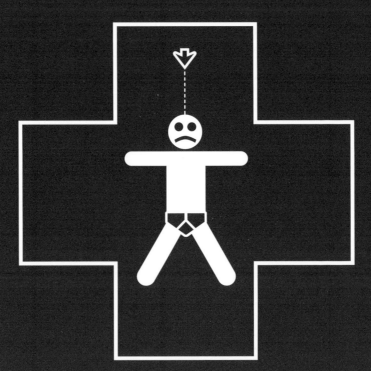

ALTHOUGH THE LINKS HAVEN'T BEEN FULLY DEFINED YET, THE CONNECTION BETWEEN EMOTIONAL AND PHYSICAL WELL-BEING IS REAL. IN MANY CASES, THE FACT THAT YOU FEEL ILL IS LITERALLY ALL IN THE MIND.

Tears of a clown

The stresses put on men to be, well, men in the 21st century are enormous. In fact it's a wonder that far more don't either crack up or hit the bottle. But the good news is that stress and emotional issues for men are being taken far more seriously now. The traditional notions of man as the fearless hunter-gatherer, aggressively protecting what is his and showing no sign of weakness or indecision are being questioned rigorously. The physical manifestations of stress or depression are being taken as seriously as any other illness, and the idea that mental and physical health affect each other is becoming central to healthcare in this country. As these ideas move further up the agenda and more practical research is carried out on how men react to modern life and how modern life reacts to them, so men are being encouraged to be far more open about their emotions, in the way women have been for centuries. Yes, it makes you feel better and will stop you taking a sniper rifle on to a tall building – it's OK for you to cry.

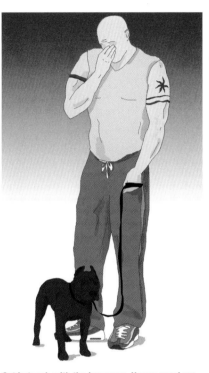

Get in touch with the inner you. Have a good cry, you'll feel so much better. So will the dog.

Men are four times more likely to commit suicide than women. The problem is not restricted to the young, either. For every older woman who commits suicide there will be 13 older men who kill themselves. If you feel depressed, talk to someone, anyone. Get help.

Dark days

We all have days we wish we could start again, or that have just been so hellish we arrive home tense, with a headache and ready to stab the dog. Welcome to the world of stress.

Stress isn't necessarily a bad thing. It is what gets us going and drives us on in tricky situations, and can be energising in ways that bring on quite a high – after winning a hard-fought contest or achieving some apparently impossible goal. But, mostly, our reaction to stress is a superfluous product of our early, woolly-mammoth-skin-wearing, cave-dwelling, Cro-Magnon lives. It's fight or flight and all the physical manifestations of stress gear you up for either combat (probably with a stone club or a spear) or simply running away as fast as you can: adrenaline boost; elevated heart rate; blood sugar surge; tightening of muscles; and

The stress scales

The most stressful events that can occur in your life are, in descending order (according to the Holmes Social Readjustment Rating Scale):

1 Death of spouse
2 Divorce
3 Marital separation
4 Jail term
5 Death of close family member
6 Personal injury or illness
7 Getting married
8 Being fired
9 Marital reconciliation
10 Retirement

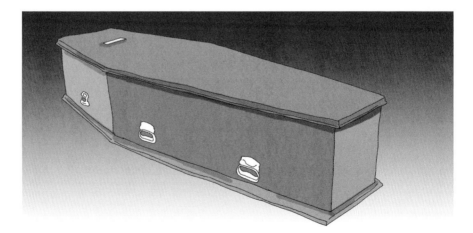

It's inevitable, so get used to the idea. But don't think about it until you're much older, or a Goth. In which case, sleep tight but remember – there's no way you can get a double (or bunk-coffin) made properly.

Money worries

Anybody who says he's never had money worries in his life is either one of the Queen's children or a liar – possibly both. Concerns about cash are the biggest single worry men in the UK admit to, and rows over finances cause far more marriages to break up than infidelity. And although we all like to imagine that a little extra cash would solve all our money worries, it inevitably doesn't – more money equals more worries, just slightly different. The key to minimising these worries is how you manage money and not how much there is to start off with.

Be prepared
Know exactly how much is coming in and construct your budget accordingly, putting money aside every month in readiness for quarterly bills.

Don't borrow to get out of debt
It might seem obvious, but to wipe out your money worries you need to wipe out your debts, so work out a plan to pay them off from your income.

Pay cash
If you are trying to keep strictly within budget, draw a prescribed amount of cash at the beginning of the week/month and work from that. When it's gone, it's gone.

Save up for things
Don't put them on a credit card and vow to pay that off, save the money by making other sacrifices within your budget. The enforced wait will confirm whether you really want whatever it is or not, and will put an end to the expensive impulse buys gathering dust in your wardrobe or workshop.

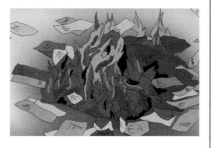

quickened breathing. Heck, even your testicles retract.

But if you've just been stitched up in a business deal, dumped by your girlfriend or cut up by that clown in the Mondeo, it's highly unlikely that you are either going to flee or start knocking people out. So after all that preparation and priming, the body's alert systems suddenly have nothing to do. This in itself becomes quite a dangerous situation. All that energy has to go somewhere and it's almost as if it turns in on itself, with the increased adrenaline and blood pressure putting a strain on the heart and circulation, the tensed muscles causing all manner of aches and pains and, for a diabetic, the surge in blood sugar possibly leading to

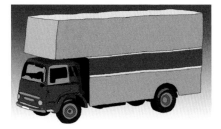

Moving house is very stressful. So take a holiday while the professionals do it.

hyperglycaemia. You may get headaches, cramps and digestive problems.

Long term, the cumulative effects of stress are equally serious. Stress produces the hormone cortisol, which suppresses the immune system, so the perpetually stressed are more susceptible to viral infections. It leads to insomnia, which brings with it irritability, lack of concentration and fatigue; testosterone levels drop; and as the muscles are perpetually tensed, sprains and bruising happen much more easily.

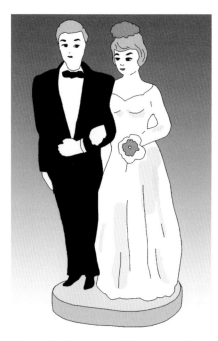

Getting married is very stressful, so don't do it unless you really, really have to. Or want to.

Ongoing stress

The most common causes of continual stress in a man's life are, in order:

Problems at work

Money worries

A bad marriage

Chronic pain – usually back pain

Alcohol or drug dependency

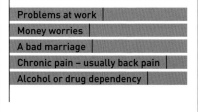

Stress: what it is, what it does

The impulses triggered by stress are of the caveman, fight-or-flight primal variety, and provoke actions within a man's body designed to help him get out of a tricky situation – you know, like a sabre-tooth tiger blocking the way down the mountain. In stressful conditions:

Adrenaline levels surge to increase the cardiovascular work rate.

A significant surge in blood sugar makes sure the muscles have sufficient energy to either fight or run away.

The heartbeat rises greatly to pump blood faster round the system and so deliver glucose and oxygen.

Breathing becomes deeper and quicker to take in more oxygen.

The bowels loosen to lighten your load ready for action.

Blood is diverted away from areas like the stomach so that extra can be delivered to certain muscles.

Pupils dilate to increase vision.

The scrotum shrinks to pull testicles up and out of harm's way.

Although we don't meet that many sabre-tooth tigers these days, these mechanisms are still triggered by stress. The effects build up within us and can have quite dangerous consequences:

The heightened pulse rate can cause a dangerous surge in blood pressure, which could lead to a heart attack.

Increased blood sugar can bring on a diabetic's hyperglycaemic attack.

Loosened bowels – never good.

Reduced blood supply to the stomach leads to increased acid production and possibly intestinal disorders or even peptic ulcers.

The adrenaline surge and rapid breathing (hyperventilation) can bring on a panic attack or deep feelings of fear or anxiety.

Rapidly increased cardiovascular activity can cause dizziness or headaches.

Increased adrenaline levels will make concentration or relaxation very difficult.

Coping with stress

When stress strikes it's impossible to avoid the physical effects, so the only way to steer clear of them is not to get stressed in the first place.

Without having to face such everyday dangers as marauding wolves, the most likely cause of stress in our lives is frustration. Frustration can be caused by any number of things, which fall into two broad categories. First, there are the one-off situations: getting overtaken on the slip road; being told you haven't got that promotion; your team losing a big game; having an argument with your wife. Then there are the sustained, progressive situations: having too much to do at work and feeling you're not coping; a family member in some sort of trouble that you can do nothing about; a chronic illness that affects your day-to-day life. Each situation needs to be approached in a different way to prevent the effects of stress damaging your mental or physical

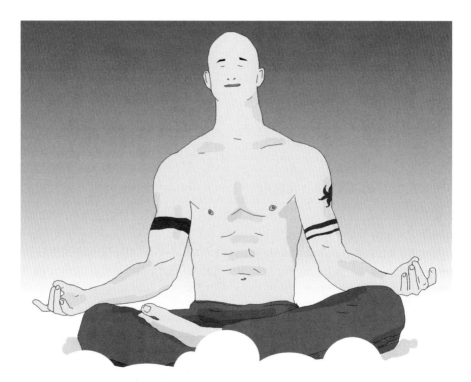

As the King once sang so eloquently, 'Yoga is as yoga does'. If it was good enough for Elvis, it's got to be good for you, so get into a lotus position and hum 'Om'.

Get some sleep

We spend roughly one-third of our lives asleep, yet 40 per cent of us say we don't sleep properly. No wonder we're stressed out.

Most men need around seven hours sleep a night, although this may vary from as much as nine to as little as five. Whatever your requirements, if you don't get them you will not be able to function as efficiently as you should. Even one night's bad sleep can take two or three days to recover from. Not sleeping properly is a major cause of stress, as without enough rest the brain and body cannot repair themselves and recharge hormone levels needed to take on the next day with maximum effectiveness (80 per cent of fatal car accidents involve lack of sleep). This can become a vicious circle, as high stress levels contribute hugely to lack of sleep. Ironically, many men admit to not sleeping properly because they're worrying about not sleeping properly!

Getting a decent night's sleep is probably the first step you can make in taking tighter control of your life and relieving the causes of stress. Once well-rested you will think clearer and have more energy and vastly improved mental and physical coordination. Yes, things really will look better in the morning. These simple tips will help you get that good night.

1 Keep real life out of your bedroom – it should be a haven of sleep, sex and total relaxation.

2 Make an effort to go to bed and get up at the same time every day, to establish a body clock rhythm.

3 Don't eat a big meal less than three hours before turning in.

4 Create the right conditions: your bedroom should be cooler than the rest of the house (approximately 15°C/60°F), well ventilated, totally dark – even low levels of light can make a huge difference – and quiet.

5 Avoid drinking or smoking just before bed; both stimulate your nervous system and keep you awake.

6 Make sure you are relaxed before you try to sleep – read (much more relaxing than watching TV), have a bath, do some yoga or meditation (see box, page 185), or have a warm drink.

7 If you really can't sleep, get up and do something until you feel sleepy. Lying there fretting about not sleeping only makes things worse.

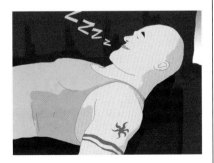

Five fun ways to relieve stress

5

1 Learn something

Join an evening class to learn some sort of new skill. It doesn't really matter what it is or how useful it will be. The whole purpose of it is to take you out of your regular life and give you something to think about that you don't have to take too seriously. Plus, it'll give you a great sense of achievement when you've mastered it. So try Italian, juggling, cake decoration, playing the trumpet ... anything that could be entertaining.

2 Eat

Carbohydrates are nature's comfort foods, rich in a substance called serotonin that can lift your mood, and they release energy slowly into your system to keep you going that little bit longer. Stopping to eat a proper meal helps you relax, too, as eating on the hoof or at your desk is a recipe for indigestion and won't give you a break. Don't fill up with quick-fix foods like coffee or sugary snacks, which act as stimulants.

3 Have a drink

In moderation. Small amounts of alcohol – a couple of glasses of wine, say – can reduce anxiety, loosen your inhibitions and help you to chill out.

4 Play air guitar

Doing something stupid and energetic like leaping around your living room head-banging to Black Sabbath can do wonders for your stress levels. The exercise will boost your cardiovascular activity and the sheer nonsense will remind you that life can be fun.

5 Hire a cleaner

If you live by yourself it might mean you can enjoy an extra hour in bed instead of cleaning up the flat, but it's more likely to stop you stressing about the mess. If you have flatmates, a cleaner will stop all sorts of arguments; and if you're married the missus is guaranteed to show her appreciation in a number of rather interesting stress-relieving ways.

Stress is a part of everyday life, but when it gets to be too much you have to act to lessen it. If you don't, you could be creating future, serious health problems, including heart disease.

health. Although we all have our own ways of looking at things, there are some broad-brush guidelines for not letting stress get you down.

The sudden explosions of stress at isolated, apparently unavoidable incidents require particular attention as these are surprises that hit you like your Stone Age ancestor got ambushed. Deal with the symptoms before they can do too much harm. Regulate your breathing to bring your heart rate back to normal and reduce blood sugar and adrenaline surges. Relax tense muscles with movement or stretching – going for a run or a workout releases a great deal of stress-related tension, and a massage can work wonders, circumstances permitting. Think happy thoughts, conjure up a scene in your mind of tranquillity and well-being. If you can, remove yourself from the situation. This is particularly appropriate if you are faced with an argument or potential fight, but includes staying away from such high-stress situations as motorway driving, a certain bar on a Friday night or ball games. And don't dwell on whatever it was, other-wise you could be heading for a chronic stress situation.

In many cases, the best way of coping with the effects of long-term stress is to learn to relax, which may involve employing a technique such as yoga or tai chi (see box, page 185). This relieves sustained muscle tension, helps you to sleep better and goes a long way to clearing your mind, so you can think much more effectively about your problems. Exercise helps an enormous amount, too, as it gets rid of tension and built-up nervous energy, and assists your body in managing blood sugar irregularities brought on by stress. Being fitter contributes hugely to your general well-being and gives you a much better chance of sleeping properly. It's important to remember, though, that it's best to choose stress-relieving activities that are non-competitive, like jogging, swimming or cycling. An intense game of five-a-side football or basketball could send your stress levels soaring.

As well as alleviating the effects of long-term stress you should also try to deal with the cause. Talking about it is the first step, not with somebody who is part of the problem but somebody who will be constructively sympathetic, as getting

Stretch away stress

Stretching your major muscles for a few minutes four or five times a week loosens you up and relieves tensions. It gets your blood flowing freer to supercharge your brain so that it copes with things better, and the increased mobility means you'll do practically everything with much less effort. Importantly, a good stretch releases the body's endorphins, the substances that relieve pain, get rid of stress and can make you feel rather good as they're the chemicals the body produces at orgasm. Develop a stretching routine that becomes a workout in itself rather than part of the warm-up or warm-down you use when doing other sorts of exercise.

5

something out in the open helps you to sort it out in your own mind. Also, by sharing it, you relieve the self-imposed pressure that a) this is somehow shameful and b) that nobody understands you. After talking things through, formulate a plan. You will feel better immediately, as you are putting yourself in charge of the situation and not being made to feel a victim of circumstances. A vast proportion of the frustrations that cause long-term stress stem from feeling out of control of your own life. Thus energised, carry your plan through in a calm and rational manner. The fact that you are now involved in your own destiny, even if you can't do much to change the outcome, will make all the difference. And this will become an upward spiral: the more you feel you are achieving the more you will be likely to attempt, lifting yourself out of the gloom for ever.

Don't worry. Be happy. Easy to say but it takes hard work to get it right. Start by dumping all the stuff that gets to you. That can include your job, your pals, your pad and even your car. Learn not to care.

Six quick at-the-office stressbusters

1 Tidy up your desk

It will be much easier to work if you haven't got to hunt for the telephone every time it rings. A tidy desk indicates somebody who can lay hands on anything he wants when he wants it and always has space to put something down. Sort out that clutter and get in the habit of putting things away immediately so that the mess doesn't come back any time soon.

2 Set achievable goals

There is nothing more frustrating than writing a lengthy 'to do' list at the beginning of the week only to find most of it still not crossed out on Friday afternoon. Not only are you likely to spend the weekend worrying about what you didn't do, instead of congratulating yourself on what you achieved, but you'll be liable to start off next week feeling resentful. Make sure you stretch yourself to some degree, just don't attempt to overdo it.

3 Waste a bit of time

Your own and somebody else's. You spend a great deal of your waking life at work, so make it as much fun as possible by enjoying the company of your co-workers. Drop into someone else's office and talk about the game or the weather or their new car or anything for about ten minutes or so every day. Don't keep visiting the same people all the time, though, or you'll start to irritate them.

4 Do things right away

If something lands on your desk that requires immediate attention but won't take too long, don't put it off because you're too busy. You definitely won't have any more time later on, so it will end up either getting rushed or not done at all.

5 Hide

In spite of the joy of other people wanting to follow point 3 and waste some of your time, don't be afraid to hide if you've got something you must get on with. Shut your door, switch your phone over to voicemail and tell people 'Sorry, I've got to finish this' – they'll understand, because they'll probably do it to you one day. It takes most people time to get back into what they were doing, so avoiding interruptions when you're busy can add what seem like hours to your working day.

6 Don't plan too far ahead

This goes along with point 2, and it will help you enormously when it comes to prioritising what you need to do if you're not worrying about things scheduled to happen a long time into the future.

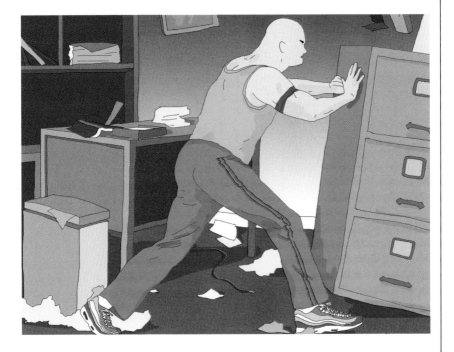

Say goodbye to Mr Angry

Everybody gets angry every so often – it's a perfectly natural emotion – but there's nothing understandable about losing control.

Anger is often the end-product of the flight-or-fight response your body produces in the face of extreme stress. An explosion of rage when faced with something suddenly stressful – aggressive behaviour from another, a driving incident, an unfair decision taken against you – is an understandable expression of frustration that helps to release the surge of energy produced. When you can't control that energy and your rage becomes a problem for other people, you have to start addressing your actions. Rage can take the form of physical violence, verbal assault, vandalism or psychological bullying, and be directed at anybody from your wife to work colleagues to a perfect stranger, but it is never a good idea.

Losing control of your emotions on a regular basis won't win you too many friends. Even if people aren't scared of you, they will be wary. And it's not the sort of thing that will impress your boss either, as it is unlikely to convince him that you can make rational decisions. Extreme anger won't do your blood pressure any good; it can trigger a heart attack and the super-surge of adrenaline coursing through your system can only escalate matters.

Different people have different thresholds for 'losing it' and it's not fully understood why they vary to such a degree. Nurture rather than nature is believed to play a part, as communication skills and points of frustration are thought to be learned in childhood. But whatever your point of no return, you need to be able to recognise it and do something about it.

TALK ABOUT IT

If you have recognised something that sets you off, talk about it either with those concerned or with somebody close to you. Don't be afraid to confront whatever it is and discuss why you aren't happy.

TRY TO AVOID THE SITUATION

If driving sets you off, then take the bus; if people in the supermarket drive you mad, do your shopping online; if you lose your temper when you're drunk, stop drinking; and so on.

DON'T GET INTO A FIGHT

If you attack someone when you're in a rage you will get your arse kicked, because you have lost control and the other person probably hasn't.

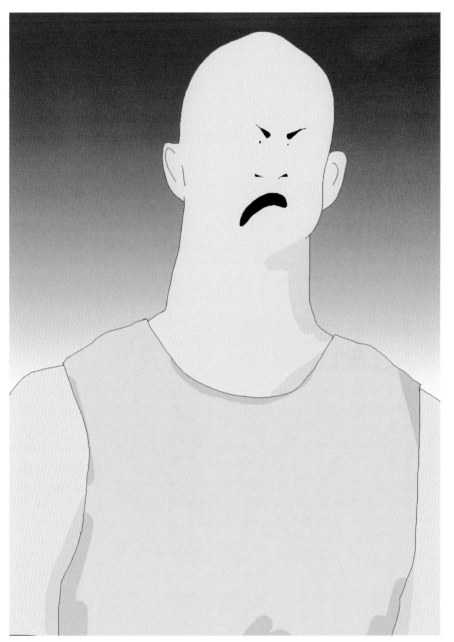

See how ugly you look when you're angry? It's not worth it, you know. Maybe you should grow some hair, too, and let it flop a bit. That Hugh Grant never looks angry, does he?

BE THE FIRST TO BLINK

Walk away from a potential flashpoint. Don't stand there seething or 'counting to ten'. Disappear as soon as you feel rage coming on, and don't worry about waiting for the other bloke to back down – losing face figuratively is better than losing your face literally.

CRY

It's OK, men are allowed to. It's a tremendous natural emotional relief.

DEFUSE YOUR ENERGY

Chop up some veg for a stew, go for a run, pound a punch bag, go to the driving range (just don't expect to cure your slice), but let that surge of energy out where it can't do any harm.

DON'T ACT IN THE HEAT OF THE MOMENT

If you do, your actions will be wild and violent and will perpetuate your rage by producing their own adrenaline surge. Also, the chances are that whatever you do you will regret later. Calm down and then plan your next move.

If you regularly feel you are on the verge of lashing out then get professional help – as soon as possible, because it's only a matter of time before you do some damage.

Don't let stress build up

When we talk about stress building up, this doesn't mean a bottling-up of feelings, but the effect stress has over an extended period of time. Do something about stress before it does something about you, because the cumulative effects of long-term stress damage you physically as well as psychologically. Stress wears away your immune system and ultimately weakens your defences against everyday illnesses. Why do you think stressed people have so much time off work? And this becomes a vicious circle, as getting ill so often doesn't exactly stop you getting stressed. As your blood sugar levels rise to fight the perceived foe but aren't expended in physical combat, the levels stay raised all the time, and this makes type 2 diabetes much more possible. In turn, this plays a part in furring up your arteries and greatly increasing your chances of heart disease. Other effects of long-term stress include impotence, peptic ulcers, insomnia, headaches and fatigue.

Relaaaaax

Sometimes it's best to put some effort into relaxing. These are good ways to get the most out of it.

MEDITATION

This doesn't have to be about finding a higher plane of consciousness. Meditation today is often used to achieve the exact opposite, as it empties the mind completely to get rid of the stresses and tensions accumulated in day-to-day life. As a method of relaxation and stress-busting this is ideal, as it allows you to unwind totally without going to sleep.

MASSAGE

Having your stresses literally smoothed away is a wonderful way to relax the body. The easing of your muscles frees you from tensions and releases pleasurable bursts of endorphins.

YOGA

The double benefit of yoga is that it relaxes you both physically and mentally, as it combines the mind-clearing properties of meditation and the muscle-loosening capabilities of stretching. Yoga goes a long way to easing muscular pains and increasing mobility and coordination, making life that much less stressful.

TAI CHI

This ancient Chinese exercise works towards 'inner peace and outer movement' and in doing so improves the body's internal energy flows. It has much the same effects as yoga, clearing the mind and flexing the muscles.

Natural remedies for stress

For the continually or easily stressed, complementary medicine offers a great deal of choice in calming, natural remedies. However, it is advisable to consult an expert before taking supplements.

ST JOHN'S WORT
The daddy of all calming herbs, it is literally nature's Prozac and contains hypercin, a substance believed to act as an antidepressant. Check with your doctor before taking, though.

GINKGO
By increasing the blood flow to the brain, ginkgo sharpens the ability to focus, reduces mental fatigue and improves the memory.

VITAMIN B COMPLEX
These vitamins can lift depression by sharply raising the efficiency levels of the brain's neurotransmitters – the chemicals that carry nerve signals. Can have a significant effect on mood.

CALCIUM AND MAGNESIUM
As well as helping the neurotransmitters function, these minerals relax the muscles.

CELERY JUICE
High in vitamin B and magnesium, celery juice lowers blood pressure and can lift minor depression or alleviate anxiety.

KOLA NUT
This was one of the original ingredients of Coca-Cola. It stimulates the adrenal glands to leave you feeling energised and it lifts the spirits.

VALERIAN ROOT
A good herb to help you get to sleep quickly. Valerian has a sedative effect on the nervous system that calms you down.

CHAMOMILE
A very mild sedative, chamomile has a calming effect without actually putting you to sleep.

NUTMEG
This works like valerian root, but not so quickly. Nutmeg takes several hours to have a full effect, so a drink topped with nutmeg just before you go to bed won't be much use. It has to be very freshly ground or grated as once it is exposed to the air it quickly loses its properties.

KAVA-KAVA ROOT
Not unlike alcohol, kava-kava works to depress the nervous system and reduce feelings of anxiety or stress. It also relaxes the muscles.

BANANAS
Containing complex carbohydrates and rich in potassium, bananas are an ideal stress-busting, energy-providing snack to have instead of sweets or biscuits during the day.

Blue, brother?

Roughly one man in ten suffers a bout of depression at some stage in his life. Only about two-thirds of those affected actually realise what is wrong and less than half of them seek help.

Depressive illness is far more common than we like to believe. It tends to strike men between the ages of 30 and 50, many of whom do nothing about it and can't even talk to their friends and family about how they feel. Such an apparently casual approach to what is a serious illness is largely due to a widespread misunderstanding about depression. Just as many other illnesses, the majority of cases of depression are brought on by internal chemistry rather than external circumstances. There is no shame in being depressed, although it can bring on feelings of failure and inadequacy. And it is very treatable – around 90 per cent of cases respond successfully to medical treatment.

Biological depressive illness is brought on by an imbalance of substances within the brain that control moods and affect the nervous system. Deficiencies in the chemicals serotonin and norepinephrine are particularly likely to lead to depression as these are mood-lifters. The symptoms of depression include loss of appetite, inability to sleep, feelings of inadequacy, lack of motivation or interest in anything, low sex drive and a physical slowing down. Any one of these can make the sufferer feel worse about himself, so creating a downward spiral as the psychological and physiological combine.

This is where a great deal of the confusion about depression comes in, as it is

Signs of depression

- Anxiety.
- Loss of appetite leading to loss of weight.
- Insomnia, particularly waking in the early hours and being unable to get back to sleep.
- Irritability.
- A fatigue that leads to slower movement and thought patterns and reluctance to get started on or finish tasks.
- Lack of interest in the world around you – your job, your family, your friends, your house.
- Reduced sex drive and possible occurrences of impotence.
- Feelings of inadequacy, low self-esteem and lack of confidence in social or career situations.
- The desire to spend increasing amounts of time by yourself.
- Flatter, monotonous speech patterns.
- Lack of attention to personal hygiene and general appearance.

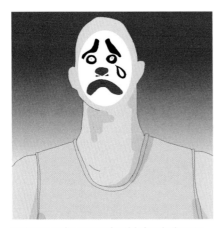

Is there a smile on your face? Is it only there to fool the public? Go, Smokey.

about themselves and, consequently, life in general.

Ideally, and in most cases, depression is treated with a combination of medication and therapy, and it usually works. But the important thing to remember is that depression needs to be addressed as quickly as possible. It is vital to seek professional help before the symptoms conspire to make life unbearable. It's worth noting that depression can be hereditary and you should check to see if there is any history of it within your family.

often believed that the symptoms themselves are the cause of the trouble. For this reason, it is important to sort out the differences between being unhappy or stressed and being depressed. However, depression can be a psychological illness, too. A traumatic experience, or prolonged exposure to a stressful situation such as bullying or violence, or continued apparent failures, can all trigger bouts of depression, and people of naturally low self-confidence seem much more likely to be affected.

Treatment for depression includes antidepressant drugs, which are usually very successful at redressing the balance of chemistry within the brain and lift the spirits after four or five weeks. Contrary to what many people believe, modern antidepressants are not addictive and sufferers are usually taken off them after a period of several months. Psychotherapy or counselling can be an important part of treatment, as they address the symptoms and allow sufferers to feel much better

Treatment for depression

ANTIDEPRESSANT DRUGS

These take about a month to work their way into the system and redress the brain's chemical balance, and are taken for several months. They are not addictive and are generally very successful.

COUNSELLING

This helps to deal with feelings of low self-worth brought on by depression and helps the sufferer to enjoy life once more.

ELECTROCONVULSIVE THERAPY (ECT)

In this treatment, which is used only in cases of severe depression, an electric current is passed briefly through the brain.

Getting to know you

No man is an island (otherwise, a lot of us would drown), and without personal relationships we would remain hugely unfulfilled. Yet it's these same relationships that seem to cause us the most grief.

When you stand back and look at it, your whole life is a series of relationships: with your mother, with your father, with your friends, with your work colleagues, with your partner, with your children ... At the bottom of every man's psyche is a need to interact with others for more than simply physical or tangible requirements and rewards. An emotional closeness to both men and women is a very necessary part of a healthy male's life – after all, it's a well-established fact that married men live longer than single ones.

Although the outcomes of each relationship formed throughout your life will be different – even within the same family or with successive but apparently very similar girlfriends – they are all based on essentially the same thing, which is how you get along with somebody else. The key to this is communication, being able to let the other party know what it is you expect and what you are prepared to give, and knowing how to connect on an emotional level – yes, with your boss or college lecturer as much as with a lover or your mother. The trouble with men, though, is that we are never really taught to communicate properly or encouraged to give anything away or put our emotions on display. You know, it's a variation of the 'big boys don't cry' maxim our fathers and their fathers were brought up with, and the situation is now complicated by the notion that modern man is expected to be more open with his feelings.

But whatever difficulties exist, they shouldn't stop us trying to put in the requisite amount of effort to keep relationships going, so that both parties are satisfied. An enormous factor in forming successful relationships is your ability to subvert the accepted ideas of 'manliness' – stuff like strength, independence, leadership and aggression – and to take a more sharing approach. This applies even to the close and lasting friendships men form with each other, as opposed to, say, the essentially superficial bonding between team mates or drinking buddies, which are associations based on much more hairy-chested notions of maleness.

Obvious as it may seem, it's important to remember that although the basics of communication are the same in every relationship, how that communication is expressed won't be. In other words, don't talk to your wife the same way you talk to your mates; don't deal with your boss in the same way you deal with your children – unless, of course, he's a complete moron. Learn to keep different relationships in separate boxes, even though the one common denominator is you and who you are. This will stop you bringing other people's attitudes and opinions into situations that really don't concern them and will greatly assist you in being honest about your approach to whoever you are dealing with.

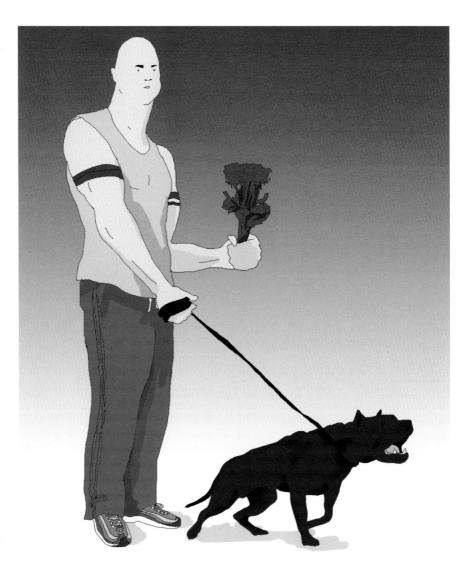

Relationships thrive on ...

Closure

If you are having a dispute about something, settle it there and then rather than leave it to hang around like a bad smell. Always say everything you planned to say and don't go to sleep on an argument.

Mutual respect

Treat the other person with the same degree of respect you would expect to be treated with yourself.

Listening

Don't use the periods when the other person is talking to simply think about what you're going to say next; talk to whoever it is, not at them.

Non-competitiveness

A proper relationship isn't a contest, so put aside that macho win-at-any-cost way of doing things.

Openness

Be direct rather than defensive. You are dealing with somebody you should be able to trust not to trample on your feelings or your fears if you are prepared to lay them out.

Honesty

This applies to both sides. Always be honest when it comes to dealing with relationship issues and, unless you have indisputable evidence to the contrary, always assume the other person is being honest, too. It will make you feel much better about discussing any issues.

Perseverance

The old adage about working at a marriage is very true, as any relationship worth keeping is worth putting a bit of effort into. Don't walk away just because things have got a little uncomfortable.

Appreciating the other person's point of view

Put yourself in his or her place while you are deciding how to deal with a particular situation. Even if it doesn't bring you round to another's way of thinking, it should affect yours.

Knowing when to quit

Sometimes it's best for all concerned if a particular relationship simply comes to an end.

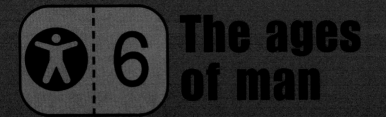

The ages of man

6

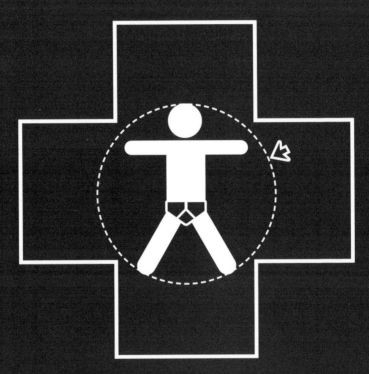

Between the ages of 20 and 70 men are in an inevitable, irreversible decline. No matter how fit or cool you think you are, as you arrange the medallion over the greying chest hair, the truth remains: you are on the slide.

Help! I'm losing it!

As you get older, your metabolism progressively burns more carbohydrate for energy in relation to fat. Not only does the unconsumed fat collect attractively around your middle, but the older you are the harder you have to exercise just to achieve the same results.

Further to this, you need decreasing amounts of calories to get you through the day – a man in his 40s requires about 3000, but a man in his 60s needs nearer 2500 – and the chances are, out of habit, you're still eating like a younger man and piling on the weight.

Your production of testosterone, the male hormone that promotes growth and sex drive, has been in decline since you were a teenager (output from the testes goes down by approximately one per cent a year from

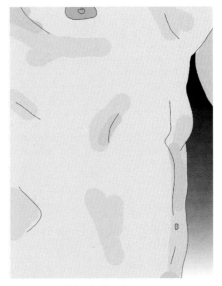

If you want this kind of hard six-pack, you have to ease off on the other, tin-kind.

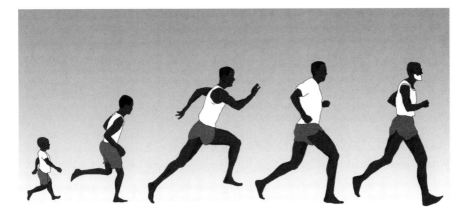

That's not a fair race, is it? That baby will never catch the fit guy. The one with the beard's doing pretty well for an old man, though. (Actually, it's the ascent of man, in the style of Nike.)

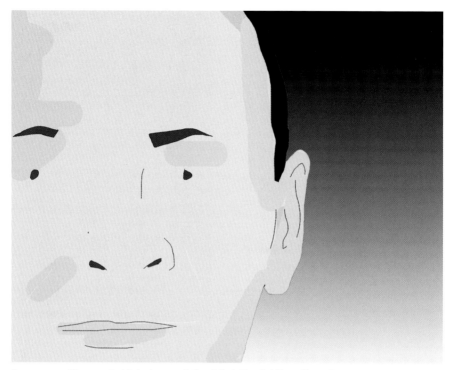

As you grow older, you start to look more distinguished. Your hairline will recede and turn grey around the edges. Just keep telling yourself that it makes you more handsome.

when you are about 20), so it's now hitting an all-time low.

You are much more prone to viral infections and illness in general because your immune system has been slowly packing up since its peak in your early twenties. By the time you pick up your bus pass it will be about 40 per cent less efficient than it once was.

Your hearing ability starts to decline from when you are in your thirties. The higher end of the sound register stops, er, registering first.

Whether you were short-sighted or long-sighted in your younger days, your eyesight starts to weaken noticeably when you are in

your forties as your eyes become less flexible. It is around then that most men start to need reading glasses.

An old man can have just over half the lung capacity he did when he was young, as the lung tissues harden up with age and lose their ability to expand so far with every breath you take.

If you had high blood pressure when you were young, you are much more prone to it as you get old. Your blood vessels become rigid with age and as a result will be far more resistant to the blood being pumped through if anything happens to quicken up your circulation.

Muscle mass declines, which is why your skin has started sagging, especially around your shoulders. With this comes a decrease in strength, and a sedentary seventy year old has only about 60 per cent of the muscle strength he had 20 years previously; this will be especially noticeable in the big muscles of the legs, shoulders and chest.

The only good thing about this decline is that you need progressively less sleep as you get older. By the time you've reached old age you can get by on little more than five hours a night, which is around two-thirds of the eight hours plus you needed as a 20 year old. But even this is no good, as with your failing eyesight, your stiff joints, your non-existent sex drive and the failing memory, there's not really a great deal you can do that's any fun.

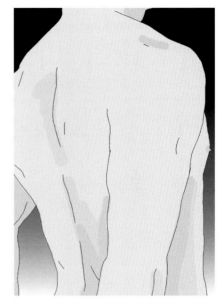

Unless you keep up with the weight lifting and regular exercise, your muscle tone will sag ...

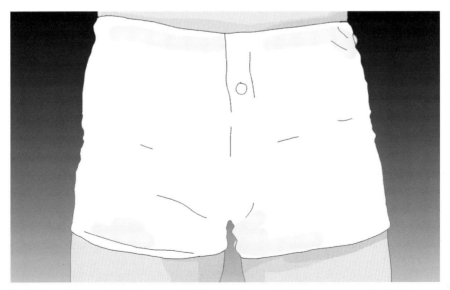

Trouble down below can begin at any age, but it is generally accepted that a young man should not wear tight, brief-like underwear. They look terrible and girls won't like it.

Twentysomething man

The best years of your life? Could be, but they're also the most potentially dangerous.

If you are in your twenties then you'll be wanting your breakfast. At this stage of your life it really is the most important meal of the day, as for most of this decade your metabolism is running off the dial and burning calories like a power station. Your body is still growing, so you're still eating like you did as a teenager with a daily requirement of 4000 calories – nearly twice what your father needs. As the need for a constant calorific intake means you'll be perpetually grazing on snacks, it's absolutely vital to start the day with a good breakfast of slow-release complex carbohydrates (see page 108). But the good news is that, despite the amount you're eating, at this age you are least likely to put on weight.

Better than that, you are at your most potent during your twenties. Your sperm count is approaching peak levels; your muscles are at their strongest for their natural size; your immune system is functioning at its most efficient (at the start

of your twenties, that is) so the likelihood of infection or illness is at an all-time low. During these years, your testosterone production hits a peak, too, so in some respects you are at your manliest at this time of your life – which, unfortunately, can have serious drawbacks.

All that testosterone and macho-ness has a downside in that young men in their twenties are more likely to die from misadventure – accidents – than any other age group. Incidences of binge-drinking are highest among these guys, and so is the likelihood of regularly taking illegal drugs. Twentysomethings are more likely to hurt each other, as a vast proportion of seemingly random acts of violence, the sort of blood-soaked shenanigans that go on in city streets after closing time on weekends, involve young men between the ages of 17 and 27.

They are more likely to do themselves harm, too. Suicide is the second most common cause of death in men under the age of 25. This is because of the imbalance

At this age, you probably think that life is all sex, drugs and rock'n'roll. Well, it might be, but you should maybe stop and think about Keith Richard here for a moment. Now ask yourself, is that how you want to end up?

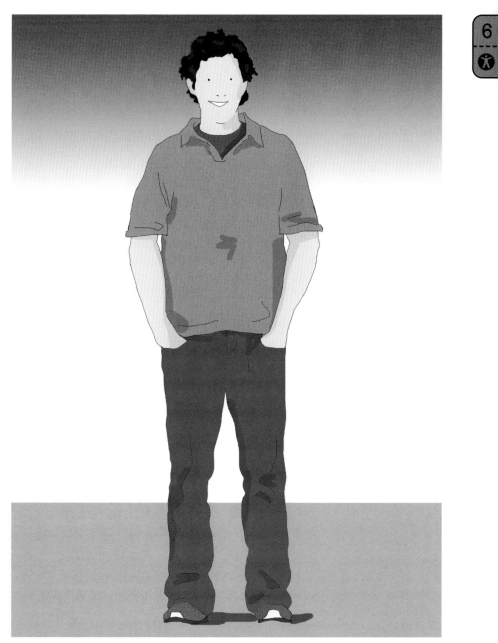

Young, dumb and full of the joys of life. In your twenties you think that you have it all. But where's the experience, eh? Live and learn, my son.

Risky business

Most of the dangers involved in being a twentysomething man are self-inflicted. While no one wants to stop anybody enjoying themselves – we were young once, too – it's worth being aware of some of the riskier aspects. Smoking among young men in their teens and twenties is going up, while it is going down among the forty-pluses. Drug usage is at its most reckless, which is to say that while older men may smoke dope and can afford more cocaine, they are liable to have a better understanding of the effects whereas young guys are far more experimental. Drinking is more likely to be binge – with the attendant risks of violence and accidents that carries – than controlled. And young men and fast cars, practically any cars for that matter, have never been a good influence on each other. There is a lot to be careful about at this age, if for no other reason than later life's habits are usually formed around this time.

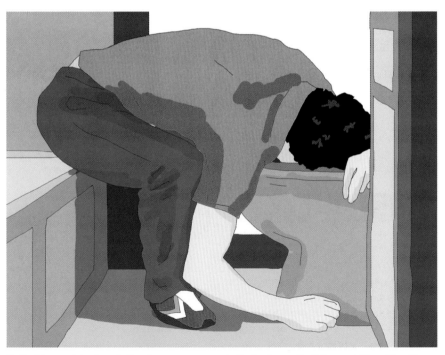

On the big porcelain phone to Gawd, young men seem to like having a celestial conversation after a big night out. Strange how so few seem to have religious beliefs, though.

between what men of this age are physically capable of and what, with their limited life experience, they are able to come to terms with mentally or emotionally. Add to this the level of expectation from people around them – teachers, bosses, parents, peers – plus the pressure they put on themselves to get ahead, and the result can be feelings of intense frustration. Then there's the question of self-confidence that affects most young men in social circumstances. They have to come to terms with a whole new set of behavioural patterns and relationship issues while still getting to grips with how their bodies have changed in the last few years. No wonder so many worry so much about what they look like and how rarely their social lives seem to be without unrelenting alcoholic lubrication.

This can be a serious matter. Boys are seldom taught to be men in the same way girls are taught to be women, and the sheer scale of what is involved in making the transition into manhood can be overwhelming. This isn't helped by the modern social trend towards an increasing number of households without a father figure in residence. Feelings of doubt are not

You should get checked for ...

Testicular cancer (monthly)

You are in the most vulnerable group, so it is vital to give yourself an examination at least once a month. If you find anything untoward, go to your healthcare provider as soon as possible.

Height and weight (every three months)

Make sure your weight isn't creeping up above what it should be for your height, and that your proportions of fat or your cholesterol levels aren't giving cause for concern. Eating habits are often formed about now, so it's important to keep a check on how yours are affecting you.

STDs (whenever you think the need might be there)

If you have been in a potentially dodgy sexual situation or are feeling uncomfortable after intercourse, then get checked sooner rather than later, and definitely before having sex again.

Eyesight (twice a year if you wear glasses)

Your eyes are still changing and need to be checked regularly.

General check-up (every two years)

For cholesterol levels, blood pressure, cardiovascular fitness, diabetes and kidney problems.

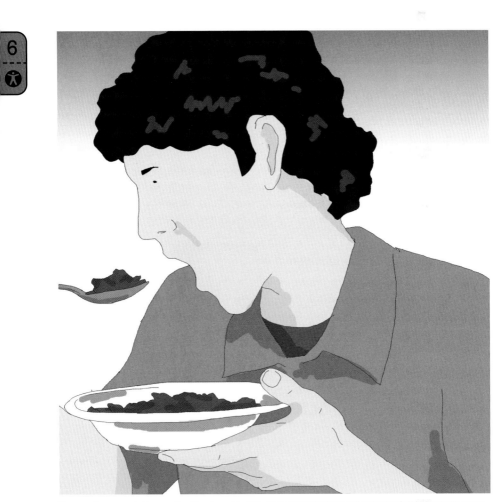

Your mother was right, you should eat your greens and especially broccoli, because it'll help you to grow up fit and strong. And eat your breakfast – it's the most important meal of the day for you.

uncommon, yet it's unlikely that too many men of this age will ask for help or even discuss their problems. Well, real men don't, do they? Low self-esteem can trigger dangerous levels of sustained stress.

The thing is for young men in their twenties to enjoy life to the fullest. After all, as well as their physical fitness they have a relative lack of familial and financial responsibility. But you should never forget you are not indestructible, nor are you alone in the world. If more young men talked about their worries and just reined in their behaviour slightly, accidents and death rates would plummet.

In the balance

PLUS POINTS

Without putting any effort into it, you are at the peak of your physical condition. At this age you naturally have a lot going for you.

Relatively, your muscles are now at their strongest.

Your immune system is at its most efficient and the likelihood of you getting sick is pretty remote.

You can eat practically anything you like without worrying too much about getting fat, because your metabolism is like a blast furnace at this age.

Your testosterone levels are peaking, making you feel pretty good to be the man you are becoming.

You've got so much to look forward to, and will most likely have fewer responsibilities now than at any time in your future life. So be happy and relatively stress free.

MINUS POINTS

You are probably your own worst enemy at this time in your life. You should be healthy and happy, but you've not got experience or the confidence that comes with it. Also,

twentysomethings are as prone as teenagers to risky behaviour.

After accidents, suicide is the most common cause of death among British men in their twenties.

You may be full of self-doubt about your appearance, your sexuality, your attractiveness, your likelihood for success ... your life in general.

Drink and drugs are probably going to be a much greater part of your life now than at any other, and so are the risks that go with them.

Loneliness is a problem as there is very little emotional contact between men of this age.

In this decade you are in the middle of the highest at-risk group for testicular cancer.

More young men of this age group smoke, a figure that is rising steadily.

Not only are you at risk from yourself but also from each other. Most apparently random violence is inflicted by men in their twenties on other men in their twenties.

On balance, it's probably not as good to be young as the young think it is and the old get wistful about. While there seems to be a massive amount of fun to be had, there are even more reasons for not enjoying it in quite the carefree way you'd like to.

Thirtysomething man

Well, you survived your twenties and the emotional and physical turmoil that went with it, so everything should be starting to come together by now. Yes and no, actually.

You should be much better equipped to deal with your life from an emotional and intellectual standpoint, as experience and progression are shaping how you look at the world. Beyond your twenties you should be far more settled into a career, making strides forward that change what you do from merely a job into something you get a good deal of fulfilment out of. You should be starting to enjoy a degree of responsibility and still have the energy to put plenty into it and not yet feel jaded. You should be a few good rungs up the ladder but still have enough to look forward to to keep yourself motivated.

On the home front, this is a potentially very exciting period when you should be forming lasting intimate relationships and possibly settling down to start raising a family. Being able to get close enough to somebody to form this sort of bond is a sign of your newly found emotional and physical self-confidence, you are able to open up and others will open up to you. Your priorities have changed and domestic bliss starts to seem a far more attractive option than going out on the lash and/or the pull five nights a week – roughly ten years of that have started to wear you out and you are instinctively looking for a bit of a rest. Now, for the first time in your life, you are able to become fulfilled on many different levels.

However, while this decade isn't necessarily as dangerous as the one before, there are two factors standing between you and any such idyll. Today's social codes and accepted behaviours allow people to 'grow up' much later, thus postponing traditional thirties developments like settling down and starting a family; and the stakes are much higher than they were when you were in your twenties.

The latter point is far more relevant to men than to women, who are keener to make the effort to settle down and are willing to take responsibility for children. Men, in theory, remain much freer and can carry on as before with their less-encumbered (so to speak) friends, who can present an attractively viable option. It inevitably leads to friction and stress within a male-to-female relationship. These days reasons like 'I wasn't ready to settle down' or 'I felt I was missing out and wanted to have some fun'

As you enter your thirties you should begin to realise that you have no idea of how to be an adult. Becoming a dad will help there – a lot.

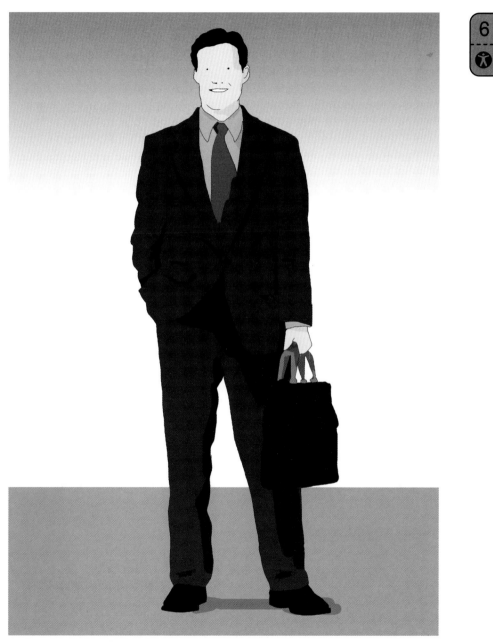

So now you've got the job, the suit, the car and maybe even the wife. All signs of maturity and confidence. So why are you still buying *FHM* or *Maxim* magazine? Because you are an adultescent.

are so frequently cited as being behind break-ups that this bears special consideration.

Life's stakes are higher because more is expected of you at this age. Success should be something you are tasting by now, not merely looking forward to, and the pressures to commit yourself to homebuilding and parenthood are even greater. In short, because you have gone beyond the starting-out phase and people feel you should be making your mark, any frustrations or feelings of inadequacy at not having done so

will be that bit more acute. It's a sign of the pressures thirtysomething men feel under that incidences of impotence are higher in this age group than in any other, except among men in their eighties.

The good news is, though, that having grown up somewhat you are much more likely to seek help or at least talk through your problems than you were a few years ago. You still might get into trouble but you now have a much better chance of getting out of it.

You should get checked for ...

Testicular cancer (monthly)
You are not out of the woods with this one yet, and the first half of your thirties is still in the highest risk period.

Prostatitis (every six months)
This inflammation of the prostate gland is caused by bacterial infection and can transmitted by sexual intercourse.

Blood pressure (annually)
Hypertension begins to show up about now and should be addressed as soon as possible.

Weight (every two months)
This is particularly important, as you

are in a prime period for weight gain. Your fat ratios should be checked at the same time.

STDs (whenever you think the need might be there)
Men in their thirties get more STDs than any other age group, so these checks are very important.

Eyesight (every two years if you wear glasses)
Your eyes have stopped changing by now, but will not yet be deteriorating.

General check-up (annually)
For cholesterol levels, cardiovascular fitness, diabetes and kidney problems.

Relationship difficulties

While being in a settled relationship and having a family can be of great benefit in terms of reduction of stress levels and general health, it can also cause as many problems. As we move on into the 21st century, men are maturing later – the term 'adultescence' for adults still behaving like adolescents wasn't even thought of a few years ago – and many are resisting responsibility for longer and having problems accepting their role in relationships or families. Much domestic conflict can result from men still wanting to have fun and live their own lives, when such behaviour is often inappropriate. Another cause of relationship anxiety during this decade is not being in one. External pressure – 'you should be settled down by now' – can lead to great stress and sometimes feelings of failure or inadequacy.

6

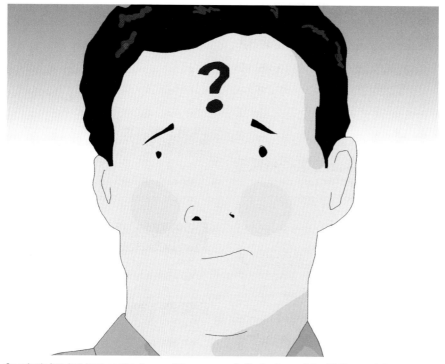

So, what's it to be? Have another beer and then move on to the lapdance club with the guys? Or leave now and go home to see your wife and sleeping child, and maybe have a warm milk before bed?

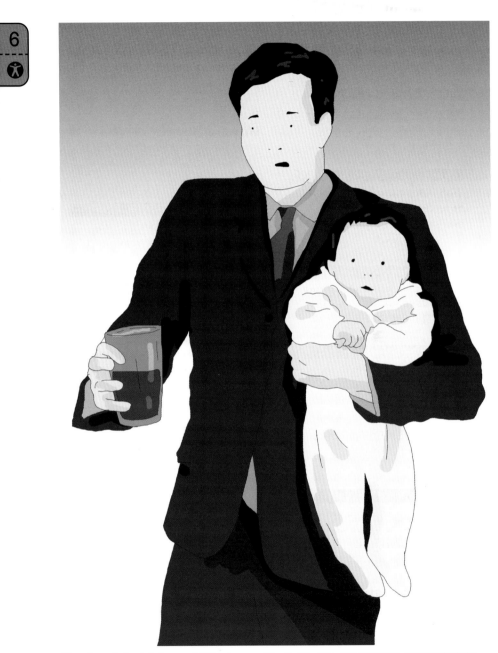

It's not easy trying to balance a fulfilling home and family life with a demanding job, playing with baby and drinking strong alcohol. Try tucking your shirt into your pants, too.

In the balance

PLUS POINTS

Your confidence levels are much greater than they were when you were in your twenties, so life in general should present far fewer problems.

Commitment phobia should be a thing of the past, so you will probably be settled into a relationship – and men who have fewer emotional problems live longer.

Career issues should be settled, removing uncertainty and allowing a progression to job satisfaction and a feeling of security.

You are still 'young at heart'. Both sexes, but men in particular, are growing up later and can carry on enjoying the social aspects of youth but, thanks to life experience and emotional development, with less of a tendency to indulge in risky behaviour.

Your immune system hasn't gone into serious decline yet, so your general health is good and your susceptibility to disease relatively low.

MINUS POINTS

Suicide rates for men peak during their thirties.

Although less likely to go binge drinking, around one-third of men in this age group drink too much on a regular basis.

Smoking tends to peak, as men in their thirties smoke more per day and are far less likely to have given up than men in their forties.

Minor prostate problems are most common among men in their thirties.

Stress becomes a big deal – it is far more readily recognised now than it is among younger men, and occurs through increased responsibilities and commitments.

As your metabolism has slowed down considerably compared with your previous decade, it becomes very easy to put on weight without realising it.

On balance, this could be your best decade as you are still naturally healthy and relatively full of energy, yet a lot of the recklessness and experimental qualities of youth have been tempered. However, it's not all plain sailing, as unresolved frustrations can be carried over from the previous decade to peak in your thirties.

Fortysomething man

Who knows, maybe forty really is the new twenty? Does life begin at forty? For the sensible, outward-looking man there's probably some truth in that old adage. Men at this age are liable to be reaching that holy grail-like balance of physical fitness, understanding of what life is all about, and emotional maturity and confidence, and they are still keen enough on things to enjoy new experiences. This is the one decade when the advantages outweigh the disadvantages to such a degree that the bad points are hardly worth talking about. Yes, you're ten years older, not quite as sprightly as you used to be and you're a decade closer to that gentle decline into old age, but the biggest advantage is that you seem to have grasped how to get the most out of life while you are still fit enough to do so.

More men get fit for the first time or mend their unhealthy ways in their forties than in any other decade. This is because it's the time when it's easy to start putting on weight, and it's when you start noticing you can't do a lot of the things you used to do with quite the same ease. And, importantly, the pace of your life will probably have slowed down enough to allow you time to do something about it and get started on that exercise programme or playing sports. These are the years when men give up smoking and cut down on drinking, too. Often, this will be instigated by your GP or your partner, but the odd thing is they've probably been nagging you for years. You can do it now because life is coming together nicely and you are less stressed, and you are less susceptible to peer pressure and don't feel compelled to smoke because people around you do. Cholesterol and other health worries have got you thinking about what you eat, too; and now it's much easier to stick to a healthy eating plan because you're probably eating 'proper' meals at home far more often. Although you are starting to become prone to conditions like heart disease and type 2 diabetes, this is balanced by the fact you are far

There has been a growing consensus of opinion in the West over the past couple of decades that a man in his forties is at the peak of his life. Yup, the baby-boomer generation has finally come of age.

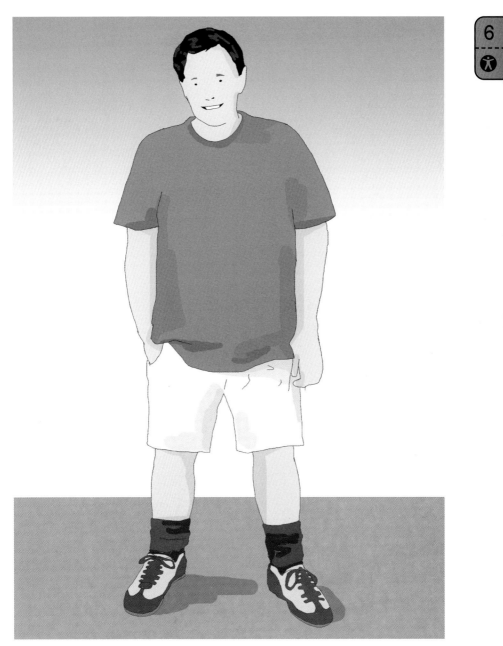

So, the big 4-0 has been and gone, and still you cling to the idea of being a professional athlete? That's OK, everyone needs a dream to believe in. (It's not going to happen, though. You do know that, right?)

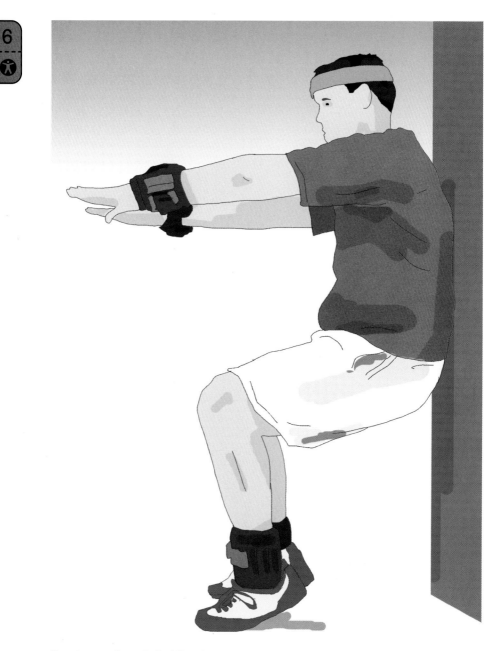

No, not a scene from a bad sci-fi movie, nor a radical interrogation method practised in Guantanamo Bay. It's just a way of telling you that you need to exercise more now that your body's starting to sag.

Exercise matters

During this decade many men start an exercise regime for perhaps the first time in their lives: running, cycling, swimming or playing a sport. And this is where the problems can come in. When starting an exercise programme at any age you have to be careful, but at this age it is much easier to injure yourself. Warming up properly (see page 136) is a must, paying particular attention to the ballistic joint warmers to loosen tendons, which become more fragile with age. Stopping when you feel discomfort is another rule that should be obeyed, and so is not attempting too much too soon. Invest in a heart rate monitor, because the purpose of your routine is to quicken your heart rate and you need to be sure that you are building it up gradually and in a controlled manner, to avoid putting unnecessary strain on your pump.

You should get checked for ...

Blood sugar and cholesterol levels (annually)

You have reached the age where you are prone to type 2 diabetes, so should check for the signs regularly – particularly if you are of African-Caribbean or Asian origin.

Blood pressure (annually)

The risk of hypertension is increasing.

Eyesight (annually, whether you wear glasses or not)

Your eyes start to go during this decade, and continuing to work or read with failing eyesight can cause all sorts of discomfort.

Skin cancer (twice a year, more if you live in sunny climes)

Any mole or growth should be checked out by your GP immediately.

Weight (every three months)

Because your metabolism is starting to slow, you need to keep an eye on your weight and body fat levels.

General check-up (annually)

For cardiovascular fitness, digestive disorders and liver and kidney problems.

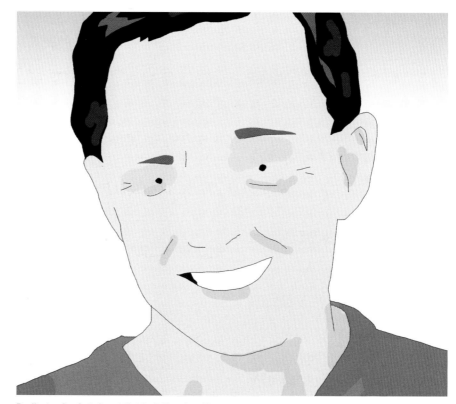

Really, turning forty is not that bad. There's still plenty to smile about and enjoy about your life. You still have some of your own hair and most of your own teeth, for a start.

more likely to do something about it, either prevention or cure. You are seriously looking after yourself.

Family life is good, too, for the average fortysomething man. The children should be old enough to be fun and do interesting things with (almost be like your mates) but still young enough to want to do them, to do what they're told and to think you and their mum are the greatest people in the world. Make the most of this, because it won't last long! You will wake up one morning to a houseful of surly teenagers and you, evil

parents, are the root cause of every one of their problems. Oh yes, and the only time they'll talk to you is to ask you for money.

Your career should be progressing, you have settled down with a good set of friends and you are reaping the benefits of the life you've been building for yourself over the last ten years – nice home, partner who's become your best friend, job satisfaction, a fair disposable income and a lot of life still to look forward to.

It may be half time, but there's still, very definitely, everything to play for.

In the balance

PLUS POINTS

Your life should be settled by now, in as much as you have a far better idea of your capabilities and what to expect from your environments.

You are more likely to be taking your health seriously and looking after yourself much better than in the past.

You should be financially much more secure, thus reducing a major cause of stress.

You are more likely to be able to talk about problems or issues, as you are self-confident enough not to worry about being seen as weak.

You should have a reliable circle of trusted friends.

Your children should be past the age at which they keep you up half the night and not yet at the age when you're up half the night worrying about where they are.

MINUS POINTS

You are coming into the lower end of the age ranges when heart disease and cancer are more likely.

Your blood pressure needs to be monitored frequently.

Juggling an advanced career and a growing family can cause stress levels to increase.

This age group is most likely to suffer from peptic ulcers and general digestive disorders.

Fortysomething exercisers and sports participants are most likely to injure themselves as they tend not to take their age into account.

You probably need reading glasses.

On balance, this is probably man at his best: not yet falling apart, still sharp enough to get the most out of life and sensible enough to know he needs to look after himself. These days, 'the Big Four-O' is not seen as nearly as old as it used to be.

Fiftysomething man

This is a bit like being fortysomething, only needing that much more maintenance.

The great thing about being in your fifties is that you have stopped worrying about much of what you used to worry about: the career path, the family, the home, the social life ... it all seems to be pretty much taking care of itself. By nature you won't be nearly so ambitious as you used to be, settling for what you've achieved but canny enough to make the most of it. Being in a steady relationship feels like the natural order of things and you are probably very relieved that nobody expects you to be out on the pull any more. The family holds no fear for you – if you've managed so far then you must be doing something right. Anyway, they'll be leaving home soon so you and your wife can carry on where you left off 25 years ago. The chances are you are very near to paying off your mortgage or it's relatively small, so

what with the kids earning now, you've got more disposable income than you ever had.

Although you are starting to wear out at this point, you could still be in excellent enough shape to enjoy this new era of freedom. If you got your act together in your forties and worked to stay fit and healthy then you'll be enjoying the results now, as the symptoms of ageing will have been kept at bay. If you get checked up by your GP on an increasingly regular basis, you ought to catch anything untoward before it gets too serious, or you will be advised on what to do to keep yourself healthy.

Of course, it's not all plain sailing. You are approaching the prime cancer-risk ages and, if you haven't been looking after yourself, then heart disease, type 2 diabetes and hypertension are far more likely to strike. It will be that much more difficult for you to get fit if you decide to do something about it

In the year 2004 the city of Memphis declared itself the birthplace of rock'n'roll. It did this in order to cash in on what it believed would be the huge interest in celebrating the 50th birthday of the music that shook the world.

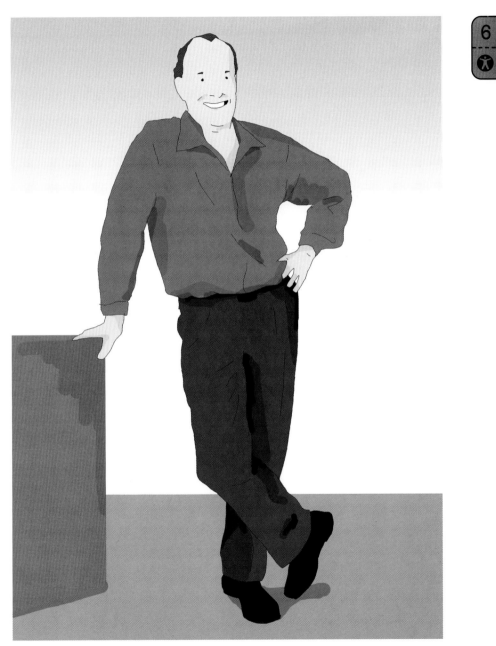

Do try not to lose touch with what clothes look good on you and which ones are far too young (or old). You should be able to afford good clothes by this age, so dress well and the world will think better of you.

You should get checked for ...

Blood sugar and cholesterol levels (annually)

You have reached the age where you are prone to type 2 diabetes, so should check for the signs regularly, particularly if you are of African-Caribbean or Asian origin.

Prostate problems (annually)

At this age you are particularly susceptible to a condition known as benign prostate hypertrophy or BPH, a non-cancerous enlargement of the prostate gland (see page 82) that rarely occurs in young men but affects approximately one-third of British men over the age of 50.

Skin cancer (four times a year or as soon as you see something suspect)

The older you are the more likely you are to suffer from this as the cumulative effect of the sun on your skin over the years is one of the major factors.

Bowel and stomach cancer (annually)

You should get checked more frequently than that if you are a smoker.

Lung cancer (four times a year if you are a smoker)

You really should be thinking about stopping smoking by now.

Eyesight (annually, whether you wear glasses or not)

Even if you already wear reading glasses, your eyes will still be deteriorating.

Liver test (twice a year, if you are a heavy drinker)

Although cirrhosis (see page 98) is not curable, its progression can be slowed down and the side effects treated.

Weight and fat levels (four times a year)

As it is so much easier to put on weight, you need to be checked for fat levels on a frequent basis.

General check-up (twice a year)

For cardiovascular fitness, digestive disorders and liver and kidney problems.

at this age – be very cautious if embarking on an exercise programme.

Also, while life may be good provided everything has gone more or less right, if it hasn't gone right you are far more likely to be affected now, as you realise that there isn't much time left to do anything about it. Mid-life crises are usually caused by the realisation that life is still unfulfilled. This state of affairs isn't helped by the fact that men between the ages of 45 and 65 are at their most prone to depressive illness.

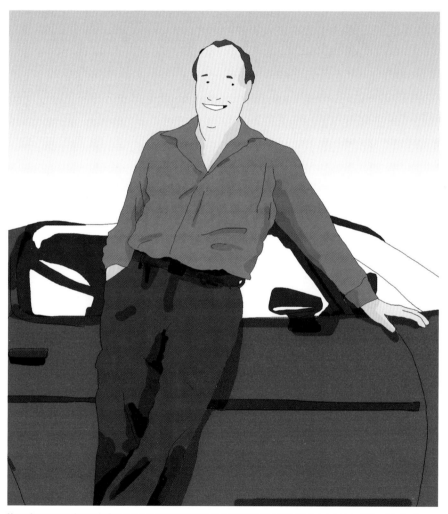

Now that most of your hair's gone, you don't need to worry about what driving a convertible with the top down, at speed, is going to do to it. So drive like the wind, Pops.

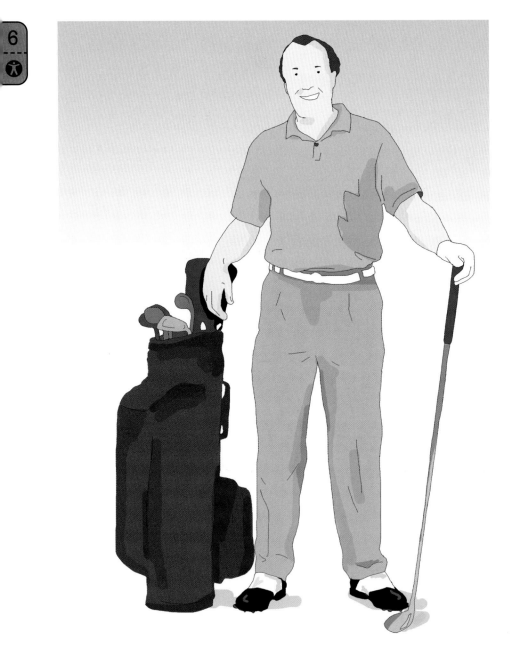

Golf. Is it really a good walk, spoiled? Or is it a gentle sport where men of similar minds meet, compete and get smashed in the clubhouse? Whichever, you've got more time to play in your fifties.

In the balance

PLUS POINTS

Your lifestyle is much less risky – older men are far less likely to suffer acts of violence, and they drive more carefully in safer cars.

A couple of glasses of wine a night are recommended, to relax you and keep your blood pressure down.

Those changes you made as regards eating and exercise are really starting have an effect, so you are probably much fitter than you were at the start of your forties.

Careerwise, you should be reaching the goals you set thirty years ago.

Peer pressure doesn't affect you, as you are liable to be living a far more self-contained life.

There is virtually no chance of you getting testicular cancer.

You have probably given up worrying about your hair.

MINUS POINTS

If you've been drinking and smoking too much for the earlier part of your life, now is when it will kill you.

Bowel, prostate, stomach and skin cancers start to become real concerns.

Your chances of heart disease have increased significantly.

Type 2, or adult-onset diabetes is a particular threat to men in their fifties.

Mid-life crisis ahoy.

Weight gain is very likely as your metabolism slows rapidly during this decade.

Your physical strength is in noticeable decline.

Your fifties are the decade during which you are most likely to suffer from hernias.

On balance, this is pretty much the same as the last decade, or at least it can be if you are careful. So, while you need to get frequent and regular health check-ups and heed whatever advice your GP gives you, there's no reason why your fifties can't be fun.

Sixty-plus man

True, you're not as young as you used to be but that's still no reason to give up.

If somebody said to you, aged 35, you could have the next 15 years off to do pretty much what you like, your mortgage would be paid off, your kids would be taking care of themselves and you'd have very little to worry about other than making an extra effort to keep fit, what would you say? Well, it's called retirement, and looked at like that your years from sixty-plus can be the most exciting and fulfilling of your life. Provided you pay close attention to your health and fitness and don't take ridiculous risks, there's very little you can't do. Senior citizens' holidays aren't just chalets in Clacton or bungalows in Bournemouth any more, they are all about trekking in Nepal, climbing Mount Kilimanjaro or rafting in the Caribbean. And, at the time of writing, they're the fastest growing sector of the UK holiday market.

Older people in Great Britain have at last worked out what their counterparts in the USA and around the Mediterranean have known for years – that advanced age need be no hindrance at all to a very active life.

The 'expending energy gives you energy' cycle has never been better applied than at this life stage. Old guys' muscles are capable of being built up to a greater degree than their younger counterparts, so being active means you are more capable of being active. Mental capabilities, too, need to be worked on at this age, and staying intellectually agile will keep you sharp and keener to carry on living a full life.

Of course, the fitness angle is probably more important than ever. You are more prone to cardiovascular disease during your sixties – heart attacks and strokes are two of the three biggest killers of retired men – so general fitness, sensible cholesterol levels and low blood pressure are vital. Cancer is the other leading cause of death, therefore regular check-ups by your GP become even more important. Maintaining a healthy diet in the face of a much greater likelihood of digestive disorders also makes sense. But staying fit and healthy should have become a habit by now. To quote the song, although the end is near, there is no reason to roll over and wait for it.

An anagram of the word sixtysomething is 'omit sexy nights'. Increasingly it seems that the anagram is funny but far from being true.

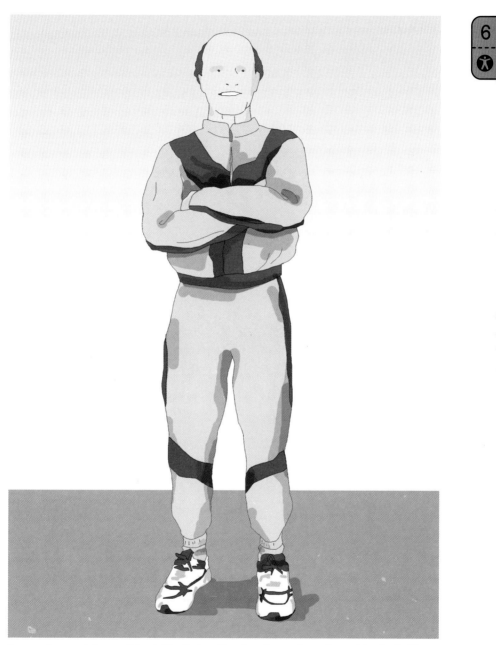

As you enter your sixties, you'll be glad for the invention of sportswear. A smart enough tracksuit will make you look as if you're health conscious. It'll also not have too many buttons to do up incorrectly.

You should get checked for ...

Blood sugar and cholesterol levels (annually)

You are still prone to type 2 diabetes, so should check for the signs regularly – particularly if you are of African-Caribbean or Asian origin.

Prostate problems (annually)

You are now even more susceptible to BPH (see page 82).

Skin cancer (every two months or as soon as you see something suspect)

Conduct checks yourself and get somebody else to look over your back very regularly, especially if you spend a lot of time in the sun.

Bowel and stomach cancer (twice a year)

You should get checked more frequently than that if you are a smoker.

Lung cancer (four times a year if you are a smoker)

If you are still smoking at this stage you are probably not going to stop, so you need to take these check-ups very seriously.

Eyesight (at least once a year, whether you wear glasses or not)

The deterioration of your eyesight will have accelerated by now, as the film over them starts to harden.

Liver (twice a year, if you are a heavy drinker)

Although cirrhosis (see page 98) is not curable, its progression can be slowed down and the side effects treated.

Weight and fat levels (monthly)

Much that could be wrong with you will be signposted by unexpected changes in your weight, so this is a crucial early warning system.

General check-up (four times a year)

For cardiovascular fitness, digestive disorders and liver and kidney problems. You are more likely to suffer heart disease, digestive and urinary disorders in your sixties, so it is vital to keep checking.

At the age of 59 years and eight months, Sir Ranulph Fiennes completed seven marathons on seven continents in seven days. He had recently had a double heart bypass operation.

6

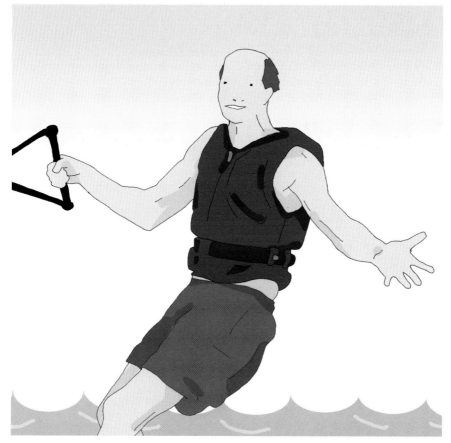

At this age you are not going to get any new life insurance, right? So go and do all those dangerous things that you always wanted, like water-ski racing, skydiving or surfing tsunamis.

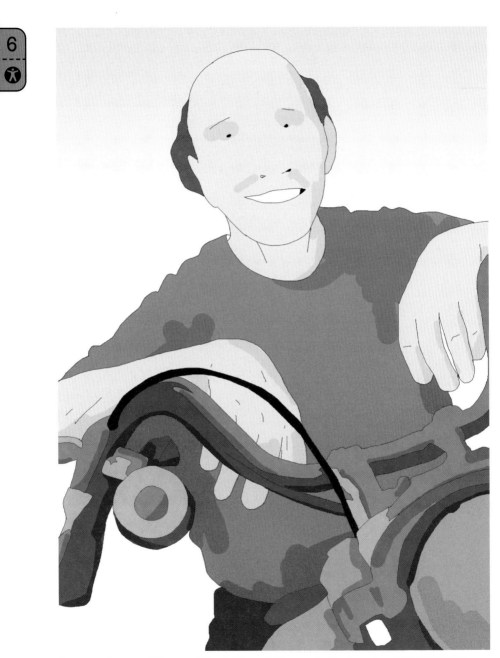

Or, you can buy a great big, powerful motorbike and ride around without wearing a helmet, humming 'Born To Be Wild' and denying that you're having a mid-life crisis (even if it is a little late for that).

In the balance

PLUS POINTS

Not so much is expected of you, so the stresses in your life are reduced and people will always be amazed by virtually anything you achieve.

Unless you are suffering from senile dementia or Alzheimer's, you are sharper than people younger than yourself because your reasoning and problem-solving skills have advanced as you acquire more knowledge and understanding during your life.

You know what is important and what doesn't matter.

Your risks of developing heart disease start falling after your mid-seventies.

Keeping fit actually becomes easier because your muscles work more efficiently – just not so hard – and their development potential is better than its been for ages.

MINUS POINTS

During your sixties you are more prone to cardiovascular disease – especially a stroke – than at any other time in your life.

Cancers of the stomach, bowel, prostate and lungs are more likely.

An average of 15 per cent of men over the age of 65 are affected by some sort of dementia, and the figure rises with age.

You have to work at being smart and keeping your mind as fit as possible by as much intellectual activity as is on offer.

You are just sort of worn out, and even if you keep as fit and healthy as you can, there is still a lot you used to do that you can't do any more.

On balance, if you've reached this stage of your life there's little left to lose. You should be as financially secure as you're going to be, your children will have (hopefully) left home and be making their own way in life, leaving you with lots of time to do all those things that you always wanted, but were too busy to do. And it doesn't matter how risky those things are, does it? Have fun!

What's the worst that could happen?

A list of ailments most likely to affect men:

ACNE Spots that occur when the sebaceous glands in the skin, which secrete an oily substance called sebum, go into overproduction. The excess sebum clogs hair follicles and traps bacteria, which multiply and cause inflammation. The condition is believed to be related to the surge of male hormones during puberty.

AIDS (ACQUIRED IMMUNE DEFICIENCY SYNDROME) A relatively new condition, having been recognised for only just over 20 years. AIDS is a deficiency of the immune system due to infection with HIV (human immunodeficiency virus), which invades the body's white blood cells. Not everybody diagnosed as HIV positive goes on to develop full-blown AIDS.

ALCOHOLISM Psychological dependence on alcohol brought on by sustained heavy drinking.

ALZHEIMER'S DISEASE Progressive shrinking of the brain brought about by the degeneration of nerve cells. It rarely strikes anybody under the age of 60, but affects almost one-third of people over the age of 85. The disease is irreversible and almost inevitably causes senile dementia.

ANAEMIA A deficiency of haemoglobin, the oxygen-carrying pigment in red blood cells. Can lead to fatigue and heart palpitations.

ANGINA Constrictive pain in the chest brought about by decreased oxygen supply to the heart muscle.

ANOREXIA NERVOSA Deliberate avoidance of eating in order to lose weight. Rarely affects men or boys.

ANXIETY Attacks of fear, ranging from mild to intense, that appear to be without reason. Can cause shortage of breath, muscle tension, tightening in the chest and high blood pressure.

APNOEA Common while sleeping (and sometimes known as sleep apnoea), an involuntary interruption in breathing that can last for varying lengths of time up to a couple of minutes.

ARTHRITIS Inflammation of the joints, causing swelling, throbbing pain and loss of mobility. The most common type, osteoarthritis, is the result of degeneration of the joints or their cartilage linings. In rheumatoid arthritis, the body's immune system turns on the body and attacks the joints.

ASTHMA Constriction of the bronchi (airways) that produces shortness of breath and wheezing. Asthma is commonly triggered by allergies to pollen, dust, fur, feathers and so on, or can be brought on by sudden stress. Five per cent of the population of the UK is asthmatic.

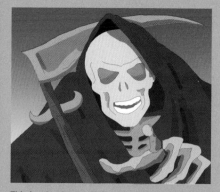

This is what happens if you don't eat your green vegetables. Death comes a-calling ...

ATHLETE'S FOOT Fungal infection that causes the skin between the toes to crack and blister.

BODY ODOUR Occurs when bacteria in stale sweat start to break down. The feet, groin and armpits are the most likely areas to cause a stink as sweat there contains a higher concentration of bacteria.

BRONCHITIS Inflammation of the bronchi (airways), most often caused by viral infection. The symptoms include a large amount of coloured phlegm and sustained coughing. Acute bronchitis comes on quickly and lasts only a few days; chronic bronchitis can linger for years. Smokers are particularly prone to both types.

BUNION Thickened pad that forms over a damaged big toe joint. Ill-fitting shoes are often the cause. Big bunions may have to be surgically removed.

CANCER The name given to a number of diseases in which there is an explosive growth of cells in one area of the body's organs or tissues. The most common sites for cancer in men are, in order, lungs, skin, bladder, intestines, prostate and stomach.

COMMON COLD Viral infection affecting the mucus membranes in the nose and throat. Symptoms include headaches, blocked nose and sinuses, fever, chills, runny nose and coughing.

DANDRUFF Flaking of dry skin from the scalp. Essentially harmless, if a little unsightly.

DEEP VEIN THROMBOSIS Formation of blood clots in deep-lying veins, usually in the legs. Brought on by slow blood flow caused by constriction or lack of movement and commonly associated with long-haul flights.

DEPRESSION Biological depression is caused by a chemical imbalance in the brain and can lead to feelings of despair, low self-esteem, listlessness and general lack of interest in life.

DIABETES Condition in which the body either produces little or no insulin (type 1 diabetes) or cannot metabolise what it does produce (type 2 diabetes). It causes high levels of sugar in the blood.

EPILEPSY Seizures during which the brain's electrical impulses operate without regulation. About 0.5 per cent of the population are epileptic.

FOOD POISONING Manifests itself as diarrhoea or vomiting caused by eating contaminated food.

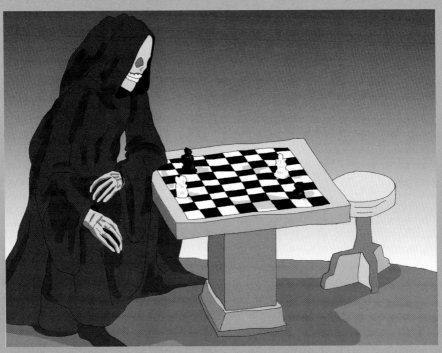

Life is one long chess game played with death. Make the wrong move and he has your bishop. Make the right moves and you get his knight, rook, queen and a few pawns. However, he will win, in the end.

GALLSTONES Small solids, usually composed of cholesterol, that form in the gallbladder. They can occasionally block the bile ducts, causing pain and nausea.

GLANDULAR FEVER Viral infection causing swelling of the lymph nodes in the front of the neck, the armpits and the groin; other symptoms include a sore throat and fever. The infection is most likely to affect younger men.

GROIN STRAIN Overstretching of the muscles running up the inside of the thigh, common among sportsmen, particularly footballers.

HAEMORRHOIDS Painful swellings of the veins in the anus that bulge either inside or outside the body.

HALITOSIS Bad breath caused by oral infection, poor dental hygiene or eating and drinking strong-smelling stuff.

HAY FEVER An allergy to pollen or house dust that inflames the membranes lining the nose, causing sneezing and watering eyes.

HEART DISEASE Includes a wide range of disorders including narrowing of the coronary arteries, weakness of the coronary valves or problems with the heart muscle itself.

HERNIA What you get when an organ or body tissue pops through a weakened area of muscle, most commonly in the abdomen or groin.

HERPES Contagious viral infection producing clusters of small, pus-filled blisters. Genital herpes is a sexually transmitted disease.

HIGH BLOOD PRESSURE Raised pressure of circulating blood, sometimes called hypertension. Clogged or narrowed arteries are a common cause and smoking, heavy drinking or obesity may be contributing factors.

IMPOTENCE The inability to have or to maintain an erection. Causes are usually psychological, but in about ten per cent of cases there is an underlying physical condition. Drug abuse, recent or sustained alcohol consumption or heavy smoking can contribute to impotence.

INDIGESTION Disturbance in the upper abdomen due to eating too much, too quickly or eating spicy food. Symptoms include wind, flatulence, nausea or heartburn.

INFERTILITY The inability to produce enough healthy sperm to fertilise a partner's egg, or to produce sperm that are able to travel far enough.

INFLUENZA Viral infection of the upper airways. Causes sneezing, coughing, aching muscles and a high temperature.

INSOMNIA The inability to sleep. A third of all men suffer from insomnia at some point and stress is the most common external factor.

IRRITABLE BOWEL SYNDROME Recurrent pain in the lower intestine together with bouts of diarrhoea or constipation or both. May be caused by stress.

LUMBAGO A general term for lower back pain due to various causes.

MALE PATTERN BALDNESS A form of hereditary alopecia in which the hairline gradually recedes as hair is lost from the temples and forehead; eventually the top of the scalp is affected. It can happen at any age.

MENINGITIS Inflammation of the brain's covering membranes (meninges) caused by viral (mild) or bacterial (serious) infection.

MIGRAINE Severe headaches, often accompanied by vomiting, interference with vision, loss of balance and co-ordination. Affects 10 per cent of British men and can be caused by stress, certain foods, or triggers such sound and light. Migraines tend to run in families.

MULTIPLE SCLEROSIS A serious degenerative disease that attacks the nerves in the brain and the spinal cord. Causes are not known.

OBESITY Excess body fat, when you weigh at least 20 per cent more than you should do for your height.

PEPTIC ULCER An ulcer that occurs in the digestive tract as the result of acidic gastric juice eroding the lining of the stomach or intestinal wall.

PNEUMONIA Inflammation of the lungs due to a viral or bacterial infection or to inhaled pollutants.

PROSTATE PROBLEMS The prostate gland is susceptible to cancer, enlargement and inflammation. In troublesome cases, the gland may have to be removed.

REPETITIVE STRAIN INJURY (RSI) Pain or discomfort, usually in the hands or wrists, brought on by a persistently repeated manoeuvre – using a computer mouse or playing tennis are two of the most common causes.

SCHIZOPHRENIA Mental illness that produces irrational behaviour and thinking and unexplained emotional responses. In men, schizophrenia tends to appear in the teens or twenties. The causes are unknown.

SEASONAL AFFECTIVE DISORDER SYNDROME (SADS) A type of depression affected by the seasons, which tends to appear during the long, cold, dark days of winter and lift in spring and summer.

SEXUALLY TRANSMITTED DISEASES (STDS) Diseases passed on through sexual contact. STDs include syphilis, gonorrhea, AIDS, genital herpes, genital warts, chlamydia and crabs.

SLIPPED DISC Occurs when one of the springy discs that separate the bones of the spine ruptures and protrudes. It causes pain, which can be severe, in the back and sometimes the legs.

SNORING Noisy breathing through the mouth during sleep, usually more of a problem for your partner than for you. There are various 'cures' for snoring on the market, but none of them is guaranteed.

STROKE Brain damage caused either by a blockage of the blood supply or by haemorrhaging from a broken blood vessel.

TESTICULAR TROUBLE Common ailments of the testes include undescended testes, retracted testes and swelling. Testicular cancer is actually pretty rare.

THROMBOSIS Formation of a blood clot (thrombus), which can be big enough to block an artery.

TINNITUS Ringing in the ears when there is no corresponding external sound. It can be caused by head injuries, ear disorders, wax blockage and continual exposure to loud noises (it is common among rock musicians).

VARICOSE VEINS Distorted and discoloured veins near the skin's surface (usually in the legs). They are caused by defective valves in the veins that allow the blood to gather in pools.

Doctor! Doctor! I feel like I'm not being listened to ...

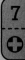

No matter how healthy you keep yourself, from time to time you are going to have to deal with a doctor. If you want to get the best out of a consultation, then these simple guidelines are for you.

Doctor's surgeries or consulting rooms can be intimidating places at the best of times. The fact that you're only there because you're not feeling 100 per cent yourself immediately puts you at a disadvantage. Being faced with somebody who appears to be talking a different language – medispeak – unnerves you even more; and when you can't read the prescription you can end up feeling helpless.

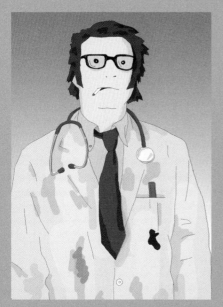

This man has the training to save your life. He also probably has a cigarette, if you ask nicely.

To make matters worse, if you have no choice but to use the overstretched, underfunded National Health Service your doctor probably won't have a great deal of time for you. This won't necessarily be his or her fault, as the average length of time of a GP's consultation is just over six minutes. This is down from eight minutes, two years ago, which shows how the gap is widening between what you need from your doctor and what he or she is able to provide. If you are paying for healthcare or you are on a private plan you won't want to waste either your doctor's time or your money, or go back for consultation more often than you have to.

Either aspect demonstrates how vital it is for you to be as prepared as possible when you go to see your doctor. You can't afford to leave any ground uncovered or to miss the point of why you are there. Besides, being clued up before you start any conversation puts you in far greater control of things and gives you confidence.

DON'T BE SCARED OF THE RECEPTIONIST

Doctors' receptionists and nurses might seem like self-appointed, ferocious gatekeepers whose purpose in life is to prevent you seeing the doctor, or at least to put off an appointment until you've got better naturally, but actually they are not. They are there to help you and any brusqueness of tone will be a result of their having to deal with a stream of time-wasters in between genuine causes for concern, and having a great deal to organise with few resources and even less time. Don't be worried about

How to get into the doctor's office

All you need is a floorplan of the surgery, an open window or two or a grappling hook. Check out all the possible entry points, make sure that they're open to you and move swiftly without running to the doctor's room. If confronted by staff, bluff – 'I'm the Doc's cousin' or 'Plumber, here to fix the latrine', should get you past them.

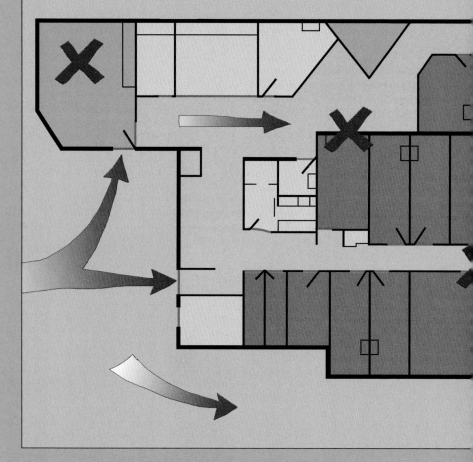

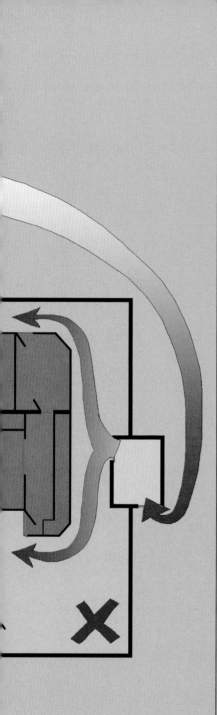

having to give a brief description of your ailment to the receptionist; this helps him or her to prioritise your needs and allows the doctor to be better prepared.

7

TURN UP FULLY PREPARED

In most cases, the first thing your doctor asks is 'What seems to be the trouble?' The more you know about said trouble, the more you are going to get out of this visit. You will be able to describe your symptoms in detail, have a better chance of understanding what you are told, know what to expect, know what you ought to be prescribed and have a better notion as to whether you are being palmed off or not. Most public libraries carry a stock of medical encyclopedias and there are numerous sensible health-related websites.

TAKE A FRIEND

If it makes you feel more confident or secure, or simply because two heads are better than one when it comes to listening and analysing, take a friend or family member with you to visit your healthcare specialist. There is no reason for your doctor to object.

LISTEN

This might seem obvious, but it's not something that comes naturally to all men. Make sure you listen to what you are being told and then think about asking questions. Ask your doctor to slow down if need be, but avoid falling into the trap of thinking about what you are going to say while you are still being told something, or you will miss out on valuable information.

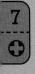

MAKE NOTES

Write down what you are told. In any conversation, it's easy to think you have fully understood and can remember what you have been told while you are still in the room, but a few days or even a few hours later it's all got a bit blurry. When you are hearing terms and discussing subjects that are outside your daily sphere of reference, it is even easier to forget. So make notes and make sure they make sense while you are still there. Ask the doctor to write things down if you prefer; he or she will probably be glad you are taking it all so seriously.

ASK QUESTIONS

Although it is totally unmanly to admit you don't know anything, this is one situation where, quite literally, your life could depend on it. Don't be shy to ask as many questions as you like as regards your diagnosis, your recommended treatment and your prescribed drugs (see panel). Refer to your notes and make sure you get answers you can understand, or simply ask to have things explained in more basic terms – you are the layman here and don't be ashamed of it.

AVOID CALL-OUTS

Doctors don't like being called out unless it's absolutely necessary. Show some concern for the fact that he or she is not only overworked but as keen on spending time with his or her family as anybody else. Unless you really can't get out of bed, find some way of dragging yourself to the surgery.

TRUST YOUR DOCTOR ...

He or she is the fully trained, highly skilled professional and you, no matter how many books you've read or websites you've browsed, are not. On the whole, doctors know what they are talking about and don't make many mistakes. While nobody is asking you to take everything on board unquestioningly, be prepared to believe what you are told.

... BUT DON'T BE AFRAID TO ASK FOR A SECOND OPINION

This is your right and while you might have to wait a while for a consultant or hospital appointment, you are perfectly entitled to it. However, be tactful when discussing this option with your GP – treat him or her with respect, and don't give the impression you have no confidence in his or her opinion. Quite apart from this being plain rude, remember you might have to go back some time soon to have your prostate examined!

ONLY CHANGE YOUR DOCTOR IF YOU HAVE TO

If you've moved away, sticking with the same doctor may be impractical. Otherwise, there's no reason why a different doctor should be better than the one you've got. Also, as neither side of a new arrangement will know anything about each other, you will have to start the relationship from scratch, and that can be a potentially frustrating situation. Importantly, though, if you propose a move within the same district health authority, don't imagine local GPs don't talk to each other – you don't want to arrive at your new one with a 'Difficult Patient' flag attached to your file! If you do need or decide to make a change there is no need to tell your old doctor that you are moving; simply register at the new practice and your file will automatically be transferred.

Do the drugs work?

The amount of illness and adverse effects caused by misprescribed drugs or incorrectly followed prescription instructions is now a matter of serious concern in the healthcare industry. To avoid any such problems, if you are prescribed anything – anything at all – by your doctor, do not leave the consulting rooms until you are entirely satisfied with what it is and what it is supposed to do. Make sure you have a clear understanding of how, how often and for how long you should be taking medication. The following points are a checklist you should go through with your GP after he or she has written a prescription.

WHAT AM I BEING GIVEN?

This means finding out more than just what type of drugs are prescribed, whether they're antibiotics, antihistamines or antiwhatever. You need to know the generic name of the drug (its medical name, such as paracetamol), what brand name you are likely to be given by the pharmacist and whether there are any brand names you should avoid.

WHAT DO THEY DO?

Again, go for specifics – ask precisely how the drugs will impact on your condition and how you can expect this to take place within your body.

SIDE EFFECTS?

Are there any? What are they? Find out why and under what conditions side effects occur. Even if they are unlikely to affect you, still find out what they might be.

WHEN SHOULD I TAKE THEM?

As well as finding out what times of day you have to take your drugs, ask why these particular times are important. It is vital that you fully understand how the drugs act.

WHAT HAPPENS IF I GET IT WRONG?

If you miss a dose or take too much or take medication at the wrong time, you need to understand what the consequences are likely to be. Just in case, make sure you know what to do if you make a mistake in your dosage and, if necessary, that people around you know what to do too.

IF I FEEL BETTER, SHOULD I STILL FINISH THE COURSE?

This is a very important question, as it is very easy to confuse relieved symptoms with cure. Depending on the drugs, it may be necessary to complete the full course prescribed, even if you feel perfectly well.

Further reading

GENERAL HEALTH GUIDES

The Cholesterol Cure
Robert E Kowalski
Thorsons

The Complete Family Health Encyclopaedia
The British Medical Association
Dorling Kindersley

The Complete Guide to Symptoms, Illness and Surgery
Dr H Winter Griffin
Diamond Books

Hair Loss: The Answers
Susan Aldridge
Self-Help Direct

MEN'S HEALTH

A Bloke's Diagnose It Yourself Guide to Health
Keith Hopcroft & Alistair Moulds
Bloomsbury

All Right, Mate? An Easy Intro to Men's Health
Jim Pollard
Vista

Ask Dr Ian About Men's Health
Ian Banks
The Blackstaff Press

The Complete Book of Men's Health
Dr Sarah Brewer
Thorsons

The Complete Guide to Men's Health
The American Medical Association
Rodale Press (USA)

Man: Haynes Owners' Workshop Manual
Haynes

The Man's Body: An Owner's Manual
Wordsworth Editions

Man to Man: Surviving Prostate Cancer
Michael Korda
Warner Books

The MANual: The Complete Man's Guide to Life
Mick Cooper & Peter Baker
Thorsons

Men's Health Matters: The Complete A–Z of Male Health
Nikki Bradford
Vermillion

Real Health For Men
Peter Baker
Vega

The Testosterone Advantage Plan
Lou Schuler
Rodale Press

The Trouble with Boys
Angela Phillips
Pandora

The Which? Guide To Men's Health
Dr Steve Carroll
Which?

FITNESS AND EXERCISE

Marathon Running for Mortals
John Bingham
Rodale Press

The Men's Health Total Fitness Guide
Men's Health Magazine
Rodale Press

**The Runners World Complete Book
of Running**
Aamby Burfoot
Rodale Press

SEX AND RELATIONSHIPS

Ask Dr Ian About Sex
Ian Banks
The Blackstaff Press

**Ask the Girl Next door: 250 Female
Mysteries Explained**
Nicole Beland
Rodale Press

The Dad's Survival Guide
Ian Banks
The Blackstaff Press

Men and Sex: A Guide to Sexual Fulfilment
Bernard Zilbergeld
HarperCollins

The Relate Guide to Better Relationships
Sarah Litvinoff
Vermillion

DIABETES

Diabetes: The Complete Guide
Dr Rowan Hillson
Vermillion

Healthy Eating for Diabetes
Anthony Worrall-Thompson & Azmina
   Govindji
Kyle Cathie

**Outsmart Diabetes (A Prevention
   Health Guide)**
Rodale Press

ALTERNATIVE HEALTHCARE

Herbal Defence against Illness and Aging
Robyn Landis with Karta Purkh Singh Khalsa
Thorsons

Index